Managing and Treating Common Foot and Ankle Problems

Editor

JOHN A. DIPRETA

MEDICAL CLINICS
OF NORTH AMERICA

www.medical.theclinics.com

Consulting Editors
DOUGLAS S. PAAUW
EDWARD R. BOLLARD

March 2014 • Volume 98 • Number 2

ELSEVIER

1600 John F. Kennedy Boulevard • Suite 1800 • Philadelphia, Pennsylvania, 19103-2899

http://www.theclinics.com

MEDICAL CLINICS OF NORTH AMERICA Volume 98, Number 2
March 2014 ISSN 0025-7125, ISBN-13: 978-0-323-26398-6

Editor: Jessica McCool
Developmental Editor: Yonah Korngold

Medical Clinics of North America (ISSN 0025-7125) is published bimonthly by Elsevier Inc., 360 Park Avenue South, New York, NY 10010-1710. Months of publication are January, March, May, July, September, and November. Business and editorial offices: 1600 John F. Kennedy Boulevard, Suite 1800, Philadelphia, PA 19103-2899. Periodicals postage paid at New York, NY, and additional mailing offices. Subscription prices are USD $255.00 per year (US individuals), $471.00 per year (US institutions), $125.00 per year (US Students), $320.00 per year (Canadian individuals), $612.00 per year (Canadian institutions), $200.00 per year (Canadian and foreign students), $390.00 per year (foreign individuals), and $612.00 per year (foreign institutions). To receive student/resident rate, orders must be accompanied by name of affiliated institution, date of term, and the signature of program/residency coordinator on institution letterhead. Orders will be billed at individual rate until proof of status is received. Foreign air speed delivery is included in all Clinics' subscription prices. All prices are subject to change without notice. **POSTMASTER:** Send address changes to *Medical Clinics of North America*, Elsevier Health Sciences Division, Subscription Customer Service, 3251 Riverport Lane, Maryland Heights, MO 63043. **Customer Service: Telephone: 1-800-654-2452** (U.S. and Canada); **1-314-447-8871** (outside U.S. and Canada). **Fax: 314-447-8029. E-mail: journalscustomerserviceusa@elsevier.com** (for print support); **journalsonlinesupport-usa@elsevier.com** (for online support).

Reprints. For copies of 100 or more of articles in this publication, please contact the Commercial Reprints Department, Elsevier Inc., 360 Park Avenue South, New York, NY 10010-1710. Tel.: 212-633-3874; Fax: 212-633-3820; E-mail: reprints@elsevier.com.

Medical Clinics of North America is also published in Spanish by McGraw-Hill Interamericana Editores S. A., P.O. Box 5-237, 06500 Mexico, D.F., Mexico.

Medical Clinics of North America is covered in *MEDLINE/PubMed (Index Medicus), Current Contents, ASCA, Excerpta Medica, Science Citation Index,* and *ISI/BIOMED.*

Printed and bound by CPI Group (UK) Ltd, Croydon, CR0 4YY

PROGRAM OBJECTIVE
The goal of the *Medical Clinics of North America* is to keep practicing physicians up to date with current clinical practice by providing timely articles reviewing the state of the art in patient care.

TARGET AUDIENCE
All practicing physicians and other healthcare professionals.

LEARNING OBJECTIVES
Upon completion of this activity, participants will be able to:
1. Review the foot and ankle examination.
2. Discuss outpatient assessment and management of the diabetic foot.
3. Describe the diagnosis and management of foot and ankle arthritides.

ACCREDITATION
The Elsevier Office of Continuing Medical Education (EOCME) is accredited by the Accreditation Council for Continuing Medical Education (ACCME) to provide continuing medical education for physicians.

The EOCME designates this enduring material for a maximum of 15 *AMA PRA Category 1 Credit*(s)™. Physicians should claim only the credit commensurate with the extent of their participation in the activity.

All other health care professionals requesting continuing education credit for this enduring material will be issued a certificate of participation.

DISCLOSURE OF CONFLICTS OF INTEREST
The EOCME assesses conflict of interest with its instructors, faculty, planners, and other individuals who are in a position to control the content of CME activities. All relevant conflicts of interest that are identified are thoroughly vetted by EOCME for fair balance, scientific objectivity, and patient care recommendations. EOCME is committed to providing its learners with CME activities that promote improvements or quality in healthcare and not a specific proprietary business or a commercial interest.

The planning committee, staff, authors and editors listed below have identified no financial relationships or relationships to products or devices they or their spouse/life partner have with commercial interest related to the content of this CME activity:
Umur Aydogan, MD; Edward (Ted) R. Bollard, MD, DDS, FACP; Jorge Bustillo, MD; Andrew N. Cai, MSc; Cory M. Czajka, MD; Samuel G. Dellenbaugh, MD; John A. DiPreta, MD; Andrew Dubin, MD, MS; A. Samuel Flemister Jr, MD; Wesley W. Flint, MD; Robert Grunfeld, MD; Paul J. Hecht, MD; Brynne Hunter; Paul Juliano, MD; Sandy Lavery; Timothy J. Lin, MD; Jordan Lisella, MD; Jessica McCool; Jill McNair; Sara Lyn Miniaci-Coxhead, MD; David Misener, BSc(HK), CPO, MBA; Dean N. Papaliodis, MD; Lindsay Parnell; Nilay Patel, BS; Nani Phillips, MPH; Santha Priya; Nicholas G. Richardson, BS; Andrew J. Rosenbaum, MD; Elaine Tran, BS; Maria A. Vanushkina, BS; Steven B. Weinfeld, MD.

The planning committee, staff, authors and editors listed below have identified financial relationships or relationships to products or devices they or their spouse/life partner have with commercial interest related to the content of this CME activity:
Jarrett D. Cain, DPM, MS is a consultant/advisor and is on speakers bureau for Integra LifeSciences Corporation.
Andrew J. Rosenbaum, MD has royalties/patents with McGraw-Hill.

UNAPPROVED/OFF-LABEL USE DISCLOSURE
The EOCME requires CME faculty to disclose to the participants:
1. When products or procedures being discussed are off-label, unlabelled, experimental, and/or investigational (not US Food and Drug Administration (FDA) approved); and
2. Any limitations on the information presented, such as data that are preliminary or that represent ongoing research, interim analyses, and/or unsupported opinions. Faculty may discuss information about pharmaceutical agents that is outside of FDA-approved labelling. This information is intended solely for CME and is not intended to promote off-label use of these medications. If you have any questions, contact the medical affairs department of the manufacturer for the most recent prescribing information.

TO ENROLL
To enroll in the *Medical Clinics of North America* Continuing Medical Education program, call customer service at 1-800-654-2452 or sign up online at http://www.theclinics.com/home/cme. The CME program is available to subscribers for an additional annual fee of USD $267.

METHOD OF PARTICIPATION

In order to claim credit, participants must complete the following:

1. Complete enrolment as indicated above.
2. Read the activity.
3. Complete the CME Test and Evaluation. Participants must achieve a score of 70% on the test. All CME Tests and Evaluations must be completed online.

CME INQUIRIES/SPECIAL NEEDS

For all CME inquiries or special needs, please contact elsevierCME@elsevier.com.

MEDICAL CLINICS OF NORTH AMERICA

FORTHCOMING ISSUES

May 2014
Common Symptoms in the Ambulatory
Setting
Douglas S. Paauw, *Editor*

July 2014
Common Musculoskeletal
Problems in the Ambulatory Setting
Matthew Silvis, *Editor*

September 2014
Psychiatric Diagnosis and Management
in Primary Care
Genevieve Pagalilauan, *Editor*

RECENT ISSUES

January 2014
Diagnosis and Management of Chronic
Liver Diseases
Anne M. Larson, *Editor*

November 2013
Pre-operative Management of
the Patient with Chronic Disease
Ansgar M. Brambrink, Peter Rock,
and Jeffrey R. Kirsch, *Editors*

September 2013
The Diabetic Foot
Andrew J.M. Boulton, *Editor*

RELATED INTEREST

Clinics in Podiatric Medicine and Surgery, January 2014, (Vol. 31, Issue 1)
Medical and Surgical Management of the Diabetic Foot and Ankle
Peter A. Blume, *Editor*
http://www.podiatric.theclinics.com/

Contributors

CONSULTING EDITORS

DOUGLAS S. PAAUW, MD, MACP
Professor of Medicine, Division of General Internal Medicine, Rathmann Family
Foundation Endowed Chair for Patient-Centered Clinical Education; Medicine Student
Programs, Professor of Medicine, University of Washington School of Medicine, Seattle,
Washington

EDWARD (TED) R. BOLLARD, MD, DDS, FACP
Professor of Medicine, Associate Dean for Graduate Medical Education, Designated
Institutional Official (DIO), Penn State University College of Medicine, Hershey,
Pennsylvania

EDITOR

JOHN A. DIPRETA, MD
Clinical Associate Professor, Division of Orthopaedic Surgery, Capital Region Orthopaedic
Group, Albany Medical Center, Albany Medical College, Albany, New York

AUTHORS

UMUR AYDOGAN, MD
Professor, Department of Orthopaedic Surgery, Penn State Milton S. Hershey Medical
Center, Penn State College of Medicine, Hershey, Pennsylvania

JORGE BUSTILLO, MD
Assistant Professor, Penn State Hershey Bone and Joint Institute, Hershey,
Pennsylvania

ANDREW N. CAI, MSc
Albany Medical College, Albany, New York

JARRETT D. CAIN, DPM, MS
Assistant Professor, Department of Orthopaedics, Penn State Milton S. Hershey Medical
Center, Penn State College of Medicine, Penn State Bone and Joint Institute, Hershey,
Pennsylvania

CORY M. CZAJKA, MD
Division of Orthopaedic Surgery, Albany Medical College, Albany, New York

SAMUEL G. DELLENBAUGH, MD
Orthopaedic Surgeon, Foot and Ankle Surgeon, OrthoNY, Albany, New York

JOHN A. DIPRETA, MD
Clinical Associate Professor, Division of Orthopaedic Surgery, Capital Region Orthopaedic
Group, Albany Medical Center, Albany Medical College, Albany, New York

ANDREW DUBIN, MD, MS
Professor, Department of Physical Medicine and Rehabilitation, Albany Medical College, Albany, New York

ADOLPH SAMUEL FLEMISTER Jr, MD
Professor, Department of Orthopaedics, University of Rochester, Rochester, New York

WESLEY W. FLINT, MD
Orthopaedic Resident-PGY IV, Department of Orthopaedics, Penn State Milton S. Hershey Medical Center, Penn State Bone and Joint Institute, Hershey, Pennsylvania

ROBERT GRUNFELD, MD
Chief Resident, Department of Orthopaedic Surgery, Penn State Milton S. Hershey Medical Center, Penn State College of Medicine, Hershey, Pennsylvania

PAUL J. HECHT, MD
Associate Professor, Department of Orthopaedic Surgery, Dartmouth Hitchcock Medical Center, Lebanon, New Hampshire

PAUL JULIANO, MD
Professor, Department of Orthopaedic Surgery, Penn State Milton S. Hershey Medical Center, Penn State College of Medicine, Hershey, Pennsylvania

TIMOTHY J. LIN, MD
Department of Orthopaedic Surgery, Dartmouth Hitchcock Medical Center, Lebanon, New Hampshire

JORDAN LISELLA, MD
Attending Surgeon, Division of Orthopaedic Surgery, Albany Medical Center, Albany, New York

SARA LYN MINIACI-COXHEAD, MD
Resident, Department of Orthopaedics, University of Rochester, Rochester, New York

DAVID MISENER, BSc(HK), CPO, MBA
Clinical Prosthetics and Orthotics, Albany, New York

DEAN N. PAPALIODIS, MD
Albany Medical Center, Albany Medical College, Albany, New York

NILAY PATEL, BS
Division of Orthopaedic Surgery, Albany Medical Center, Albany, New York

NANI PHILLIPS, MPH
Division of Orthopaedic Surgery, Albany Medical Center, Albany, New York

NICHOLAS G. RICHARDSON, BS
Albany Medical College, Albany, New York

ANDREW J. ROSENBAUM, MD
Resident, Division of Orthopaedic Surgery, Albany Medical Center, Albany Medical College, Albany, New York

ELAINE TRAN, BS
Albany Medical College, Albany, New York

MARIA A. VANUSHKINA, BS
Albany Medical College, Albany, New York

STEVEN B. WEINFELD, MD
Associate Professor of Orthopaedic Surgery, Chief, Foot and Ankle Service, Icahn School
of Medicine at Mount Sinai, New York, New York

Contents

to present with medial pain and swelling, but later in the disease process can also present with lateral-sided pain. The mainstay of nonoperative treatment is nonsteroidal anti-inflammatory drugs, weight loss, and orthotic insoles or brace use. The goals of therapy are to provide relief of symptoms and prevent progression of the deformity. If nonoperative management fails, a variety of surgical procedures are available; however, these require a lengthy recovery, and therefore patients should be advised accordingly.

The cavus, or high-arched, foot can present in either childhood or adulthood as a function of muscle imbalance. Neurologic, traumatic, and idiopathic processes have been identified, along with residual clubfoot, as the primary causes of adult cavus foot deformity. A thorough history and physical examination is important and can help identify the underlying cause of deformity. Conservative treatment modalities are always used first, with surgical intervention reserved for refractory cases. The goal of surgery is to correct muscle imbalance, which can be achieved via tendon transfers, corrective osteotomies, and, in the most severe cases, fusion.

Ankle injuries are among the most common injuries presenting to primary care providers and emergency departments and may cause considerable time lost to injury and long-term disability. Inversion injuries about the ankle involve about 25% of all injuries of the musculoskeletal system and 50% of all sports-related injuries. Medial-sided ankle sprains occur less frequently than those on the lateral side. High ankle sprains occur less frequently in the general population, but do occur commonly in collision sports. Providers should apply the Ottawa ankle rules when radiography is indicated and refer fractures and more severe injuries to orthopedic surgery as needed.

Achilles tendon disorders include tendinosis, paratenonitis, insertional tendinitis, retrocalcaneal bursitis, and frank rupture. Patients present with pain and swelling in the posterior aspect of the ankle. Magnetic resonance imaging and ultrasound are helpful in confirming the diagnosis and guiding treatment. Nonsurgical management of Achilles tendon disorders includes nonsteroidal anti-inflammatory drugs, physical therapy, bracing, and footwear modification. Surgical treatment includes debridement of the diseased area of the tendon with direct repair. Tendon transfer may be necessary to augment the strength of the Achilles tendon.

Plantar heel pain is a common complaint encountered by orthopedic surgeons, internists, and family practitioners. Although it is most often caused by plantar fasciitis, this is a diagnosis of exclusion. Other mechanical, rheumatologic, and neurologic causes must be considered first. The history and physical examination are typically all that is needed to make the proper diagnosis, but diagnostic adjuncts are available to assist the clinician. When plantar fasciitis is diagnosed, conservative modalities must be tried first. Corticosteroid injections and extracorporeal shockwave therapy may also be used. After 6 months of failed conservative treatments, surgical intervention should be considered.

Patients with diabetes and peripheral neuropathy are at risk for foot deformities and mechanical imbalance of the lower extremity. Peripheral neuropathy leads to an insensate foot that puts the patient at risk for injury. When combined with deformity due to neuropathic arthropathy, or Charcot foot, the risks of impending ulceration, infection, and amputation are significant to the diabetic patient. Education of proper foot care and shoe wear cannot be overemphasized. For those with significant malalignment or deformity of the foot and ankle, referral should be made immediately to an orthopedic foot and ankle specialist.

Foreword

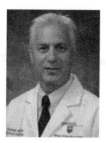

Edward (Ted) R. Bollard, MD, DDS, FACP
Consulting Editor

Foot and ankle problems are common in the general population. In addition, the prevalence increases with age. It has been estimated that 20 to 40% of older adults report pain in their feet. It is also important to note that a larger percentage of patients have conditions involving the feet that are nontraumatic, nonpainful, yet may result in symptoms and/or alteration in form and function if gone undiagnosed and untreated. Therefore, it is not surprising that a chief complaint involving the foot or ankle comprises a significant percentage of consultations with primary care physicians. In this issue of *Medical Clinics of North America*, our expert, orthopedic guest editor, John DiPreta, MD provides a standard approach to the examination of the foot and ankle complex, and the understanding of the association of these structures to gait and ambulation. In addition, the articles to follow review the presentation, evidence-based diagnostic evaluation, therapeutic modalities, recommended follow-up care, and appropriate subspecialty referral for many of the common foot conditions encountered in the outpatient setting.

Edward (Ted) R. Bollard, MD, DDS, FACP
Graduate Medical Education
Penn State University College of Medicine
500 University Drive
P. O. Box 850 (Mail Code H039)
Hershey, PA 17033-0850, USA

E-mail address:
ebollard@hmc.psu.edu

Med Clin N Am 98 (2014) xv
http://dx.doi.org/10.1016/j.mcna.2013.12.001
0025-7125/14/$ – see front matter © 2014 Published by Elsevier Inc.

medical.theclinics.com

Preface

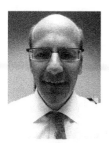

John A. DiPreta, MD
Editor

It is an honor to serve as the guest editor for this issue of the *Medical Clinics of North America*. The authors for this issue have striven to provide current reviews of common conditions encountered by the primary care physician. Disorders of the foot and ankle are a common reason for patients to seek consultation with their primary care providers. This issue of *Medical Clinics of North America* is dedicated to office-based management and decisions for referral for these disorders.

An emphasis has been placed on the initial assessment of foot and ankle conditions, gait abnormalities, and pertinent exam skills. Each of these topical reviews provides a discussion of the pathophysiology of the particular condition. Subject reviews include diabetic foot, metatarsalgia, Achilles tendon pathology, ankle sprains and instability, cavovarus foot deformity, plantar heel pain, nail and skin disorders, arthritides of the ankle and foot, hallux valgus, and evaluation of the adult acquired flatfoot. While an emphasis is made on the initial evaluation and the pathophysiology of these disorders, a review of commonly accepted treatments is made and recommendations for referral to a foot and ankle specialist are discussed.

The articles also demonstrate the complexity of the aforementioned conditions and the integral role that the primary care physician plays in the initial assessment, management, and referral of their patients to the foot and ankle specialist. The authors are indeed very passionate about their profession and it is my hope that this issue will be a valuable resource for the primary care practitioner and their patients.

I would like to extend my thanks to all the contributing and corresponding authors. Their contributions made my role easier and, without their efforts, this would have not been possible. I would also like to extend my thanks to Jess McCool at Elsevier for her guidance and assistance in crafting this project. Finally, I would like to thank my wife,

Med Clin N Am 98 (2014) xvii–xviii
http://dx.doi.org/10.1016/j.mcna.2013.10.012
0025-7125/14/$ – see front matter

medical.theclinics.com

Amy, and children, Lucas, Antonia, Joseph, and James, for giving me the time and their patience to complete this project.

John A. DiPreta, MD
Division of Orthopaedic Surgery
Capital Region Orthopaedic Group
Albany Medical Center
Albany Medical College
1367 Washington Avenue, Suite 200
Albany, NY 12206, USA

E-mail address:
jamddipreta@netscape.net

The Foot and Ankle Examination

Dean N. Papaliodis, MD[a],*, Maria A. Vanushkina, BS[b],
Nicholas G. Richardson, BS[b], John A. DiPreta, MD[a]

KEYWORDS

- Foot/Ankle physical examination • Structural abnormalities • Ottawa ankle rules
- Special tests

KEY POINTS

- Knowledge of common foot and ankle complaints can be diagnosed and managed effectively in the primary care setting.
- Foot and ankle disorders require a thorough and structured history and physical examination with attention to the patient as a whole.
- Knowledge of foot and ankle anatomy and biomechanics is key in successful clinical evaluation and therapeutic considerations.

INTRODUCTION

Foot and ankle disorders (FAD) are highly prevalent in the general population and are one of the leading motivations for primary care visits.[1–4] Unfortunately, many physicians consider FAD diagnostically challenging and the management daunting.[5] On initial approach, the goal is to establish a historical database to characterize the problem, infer the structures involved, and assess prognosis.[6] A history should elucidate symptoms, chronicity, pathomechanics, and relevant past medical conditions (**Box 1**). Epidemiologic factors, such as age, gender, employment, and activities, are of great diagnostic value and help individualize the history, physical examination, and treatment.[1] Physical examination findings should be interpreted in the context of overall health, vital signs, and symptoms. A head-to-toe inspection is the first step. Failing to expose the lower extremities sufficiently is a mistake; patients should be in a gown with shoes and socks removed. Footwear patterns provide valuable information and shoes should be evaluated for appropriate fit.[7] A thorough physical examination examines structural integrity through palpation, mobility, and strength testing. Many disorders mimic each other on initial presentation and provocative tests help

[a] Division of Orthopaedic Surgery, Albany Medical Center, Albany Medical College, MC184, 1367 Washington Avenue, Suite 202, Albany, NY 12206, USA; [b] Albany Medical College, MC184, 1367 Washington Avenue, Suite 202, Albany, NY 12206, USA
* Corresponding author.
E-mail address: papalid@mail.amc.edu

Med Clin N Am 98 (2014) 181–204
http://dx.doi.org/10.1016/j.mcna.2013.10.001
0025-7125/14/$ – see front matter © 2014 Elsevier Inc. All rights reserved.

Box 1
Suggested historical evaluation

What are your goals regarding functional results after treatment?

Symptoms

  Describe pain: Location, duration, radiation, intensity, and type

  Describe swelling: chronicity, location, duration, color changes

  Any new muscle weakness? Atrophy? Numbness, tingling, or burning?

  Any foot or ankle instability? Feeling of giving way?

  Have you tried rest, ice, compression, elevation, medications, hot packs?

  What exacerbates symptoms?

  How are the symptoms affected by physical activity? Rest?

  Have you received any therapy for this injury? How much time passed since the onset before you sought treatment? Why seek treatment now?

  What activities have you been able to do since onset? Affecting activities of daily living?

Mechanism of injury

  What type of activity lead to this injury?

  How often and for how long do you engage in this activity?

  If traumatic, describe mechanism: trip, fall, twist ankle, etc

  What do you think happened? Did you injure anything else?

  Did you have any sensation of popping or cracking at the time?

  Were you able to walk (even with a limp) immediately after the injury?

Chronicity

  Onset: acute, gradual, traumatic versus nontraumatic? Is this a recurrence?

  Describe symptom progression over time.

  Symptom severity correlated with time? AM, PM, activity?

Social history

  What do you do for work? Does it involve physical activity?

  What type of regular exercise do you perform?

  Have you had changes in your activity level over the past 6 months: duration, intensity, frequency, or equipment?

  What type of shoes do you wear? How often do you change them?

  Describe substance use: Tobacco/alcohol especially

Past medical history

  Prior back, extremity injuries or disorders? When? Treatment?

  History of diabetes/vascular disease? See a podiatrist?

  Other endocrine, coagulation, vascular, systemic inflammatory, neuromuscular, nutritional, kidney, or arthritic disorders?

  Current medications? For what conditions? Recent antibiotic use?

  Any past imaging studies? X-ray, CT, MRI, US

  Are you up-to-date on immunizations? Last tetanus shot?

Data from Boulton AJ, Armstrong DG, Albert SF, et al. Comprehensive foot examination and risk assessment: a report of the task force of the foot care interest group of the American Diabetes Association, with endorsement by the American Association of Clinical Endocrinologists. Diabetes Care 2008;31(8):1679–85.

differentiate similar or coexisting conditions.[8] Evaluation should be performed in multiple positions, such as walking, standing, seated, and prone. The unaffected extremity should be used as a reference point for all examination findings. Many problems do not require specialist referral and can be managed with protection, relative rest, ice, compression, elevation, medications, or rehabilitation modalities (PRICEMR).[9,10]

SKIN EXAMINATION

Skin integrity should be assessed first. Hyperkeratotic lesions such as calluses and corns can frequently form in areas of increased friction and pressure.[1] Diabetes, obesity, structural abnormalities, and poorly fitting shoes are common conditions associated with increased pressure.[11] In diabetic feet, these pressure points can become sites of future ulceration. Aside from calluses, there are several common soft tissue alterations in diabetic feet: increased thickness of plantar fascia, decreased thickness of plantar soft tissue, accentuated hardness of the overlying skin, and a propensity for ulcer formation.[12] Ulcers may be hidden by the overlying hyperkeratosis, which should be debrided to relieve pain and allow proper assessment.[13]

Infections

Superficial conditions, such as tinea pedis, plantar warts, pitted keratolysis, and onychomycosis, are obvious on inspection and eventually resolve on their own in healthy patients but targeted topical treatments are often more expedient.[14] Cellulitis and erysipelas are common infections of the dermis and underlying soft tissue structures. Both present as obviously red, hot, swollen, and tender expanses often without any obvious breach in skin integrity. Poorly demarcated margins versus raised borders and burning pain distinguish cellulitis from erysipelas. Normal skin flora such as *Staphylococcus* or group A *Streptococcus* are the most common pathogens and are best treated with empiric oral antibiotics, ibuprofen, and elevation. Purulent cellulitis should be empirically covered for methicillin-resistant *Staphylococcus aureus* pending culture and sensitivity. Cutaneous abscesses should be drained.[15] Further studies are not required unless there are signs of systemic toxicity or high suspicion for deep infections.[14]

In the setting of any localized inflammation around a joint, septic arthritis should be high on the differential. Joint sepsis is present in one-third of osteomyelitis cases.[16] Adult patients should be assessed for predisposing factors, such as diabetes, cirrhosis, cancer, traumatic joint damage, surgery, hemoglobinopathies, corticosteroids or immunosuppressants, HIV/AIDS, chronic joint disease, and alcohol and intravenous drug abuse.[17] Signs of systemic infection, such as fever or lethargy, multiple joint involvement, abnormal gait, limited range of motion (ROM), tenderness, skin lesions, and ulcers, should be assessed during a physical examination. Workup includes arthrocentesis, blood cultures, Gram stains, erythrocyte sedimentation rate, and plain films.[16] Septic arthritis is more common in all children and is often unprovoked.[18] Physicians should maintain high clinical suspicion for osteomyelitis of adjacent bones. Osteomyelitis in children is classically thought to affect the metaphyseal regions of long bones; however, a recent study found that bones of the foot are actually most commonly involved.[19] Bone biopsies are the gold standard for diagnosis.

Diabetic feet are especially susceptible to all infections. Dry skin with cracks and fissures provides easy access to infections that progress rapidly without an adequate immune system and vascular supply.[12] There is a 15% lifetime chance of developing a foot infection in this population.[14] Infections are frequently coincident with ulcers, but one is not necessary for the presence of the other. Foot ulceration is the most significant risk factor for amputation. Most nontraumatic amputations occur in diabetic patients and are preventable with vigilant screening (**Table 1**).[7] For patients with existing ulcers, the likelihood and severity of infection increase with any of the following features: lesions measuring greater than 2 cm, grossly exposed or palpable bone at ulcer site, erythrocyte sedimentation rate greater than 70 mm/h, and corroborating radiologic abnormalities.[14]

STRUCTURAL ABNORMALITIES

Congenital and acquired variation in lower extremity form is common. In children, intoeing and flatfeet (FF) are especially prevalent structural disorders seen in the first decade of life; both are usually asymptomatic, improve naturally with age, and have a strong genetic component.[20] Parents report a family history of the condition and will worry about the psychosocial and functional implications of the deformity and its treatment on the child.[20] In most cases, reassurance is the only intervention necessary. In adults, arch and digital deformities prevail and are more likely to be pathologic and painful and lead to significant morbidity. Between 5% and 20% of adults have FF and more than one-third of adults will develop a digital deformity, such as hallux valgus (HVD).[21,22] Unlike childhood abnormalities, adult-onset structural disorders can be disabling and often require medical or surgical intervention.

Arch Disorders

FF have numerous causes; classification according to age of onset and foot flexibility is the most informative for prognosis and treatment. Pediatric FF are present before skeletal maturity and adult FF are present after. Flexible flatfeet (FFF) retain a normal arch while in a dependent position and flatten on standing.[23] Rigid flatfeet are

Table 1 Diabetic foot screening guidelines		
Ulcer Risk Factors	**Historical Features**	**Essential Physical Examination**
PN	Past medical history:	Inspection
Foot deformity	Ulceration, amputation,	Skin
Foot trauma	Charcot joint, vascular	Color, thickness, dryness, cracking;
Previous amputation	surgery, angioplasty,	sweating; infection (check
Past foot ulcer history	cigarette smoking	between toes for fungal);
Peripheral vascular	Neuropathic symptoms:	ulceration; calluses/blistering
disease	Burning, shooting, pain,	(hemorrhage into callus?)
Visual impairment	electrical, or sharp	Musculoskeletal
Diabetic nephropathy	sensations	Deformity, such as claw toes,
Poor glycemic control	Numbness, dead feet	prominent metatarsal heads,
Cigarette smoking	Vascular symptoms:	Charcot joint, HVD; muscle wasting
	Claudication, rest pain,	(guttering between metatarsals)
	nonhealing ulcer	Neurologic assessment
	Other complications:	10-g monofilament + 1 of the
	Renal, retinal	following 4: Vibration using 128-Hz
		tuning fork; pinprick sensation; ankle
		reflexes; vibration perception
		threshold testing
		Vascular assessment
		Foot pulses (ABI if indicated)

Data from Rogers LC, Frykberg RG, Armstrong DG, et al. The Charcot foot in diabetes. Diabetes Care 2011;34(9):2123–9.

characterized by a stiff, flattened arch on and off weight-bearing.[20] On inspection, patients will have at least one of the following: forefoot supination, a depressed medial arch, medial talar head prominence, hindfoot eversion, and a positive Helbing sign, which is described as medial or inward deviation of the Achilles tendon (**Fig. 1**).[22] More than the normal 1 to 2 toes will be visible on the lateral border when looking from behind (see **Fig. 1**), referred to as the "too many toes sign."[24] Single leg heel raises (SHR) and Jack's toe raises are diagnostic tests that look for reconstitution of the arch.[20] SHR is observed from behind with the patient's hands against a wall for support.[24] On single toe standing, normal feet and FFF will have heel inversion and a visible arch (**Fig. 2**). Patients with normal subtalar joint motion and plantar flexor strength are able to perform at least 10 SHR on each side. Jack's toe raises uses the same "windlass mechanism" as SHR. With the patient standing, the hallux is passively extended to create an arch (**Fig. 3**).[22]

Digital Deformities

HVD is a heritable progressive deformity presenting with abduction and valgus rotation of the great toe and a medially prominent first metatarsal head.[25] HVD is the most common digital deformity with a prevalence of 23% in adults aged 18 to 65 years.[21] The prevalence is estimated at 35.7% in the elderly, where it increases gait instability and fall risk.[21,26] Even severe deformities may be asymptomatic; however, many patients with will report high self-perceived disability.[27] Pain is usually

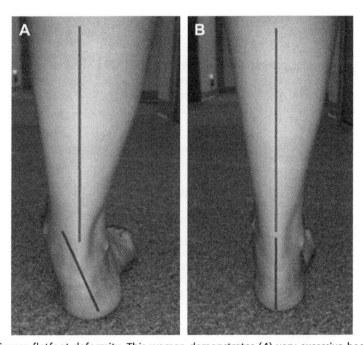

Fig. 1. Severe flatfoot deformity. This woman demonstrates (A) very excessive heel valgus and the lateral bow of the tendo-Achilles known as the positive Helbing sign as well as excessive toes visible on the lateral border known as the Too Many Toes sign; (B) the classic medial collapse of the foot; and retained ability to perform a double heel raise, but a marked lack of supinatory varus in the heel. (*From* Lee MS, Vanore JV, Thomas JL, et al. Diagnosis and treatment of adult flatfoot. J Foot Ankle Surg 2005;44(2):78–113; with permission.)

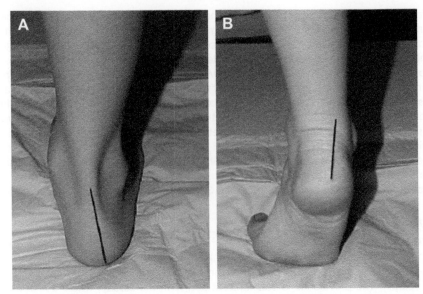

Fig. 2. Examination of hindfoot movement. In normal feet as well as in patients with flexible flatfoot, the valgus heel (*A*) in stance changes to a varus (*B*) position with the clinical maneuver of SHR, showing the flexible nature and the reducibility of the deformity. (*From* Harris EJ, Vanore JV, Thomas JL, et al. Diagnosis and treatment of pediatric flatfoot. J Foot Ankle Surg 2004;43(6):341–73; with permission.)

associated with inflammation of the overlying soft tissue structures exacerbated by inappropriately fitting footwear,[13] usually referred to as a bunion. There are multiple associated conditions such as hammer toes, calluses under the second metatarsal, metatarsal pain, and ingrown toenails. ROM at the first metatarsophalangeal (MTP)

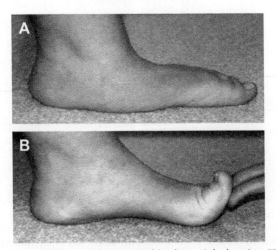

Fig. 3. Jack's toe raise test (*A*). An arch is created in the weight-bearing FFF by the windlass action of the great toe and the plantar fascia (*B*). (*From* Evans AM. The pocket podiatry guide: pediatrics. Edinburgh (Scotland): Churchill Livingstone; 2010. p. 107–37; with permission.)

joint, normally confined exclusively to the sagittal plane, may include oblique deviation such as abduction and eversion during dorsiflexion.[25] To test hallux ROM, the midfoot is stabilized with one hand and the other is used to extend and flex the great toe maximally. The MTP joint is capable of 0° to 70° of extension and 0° to 45° of flexion.[28] Loss of motion, most significantly extension, in the MTP is critical and results in an abnormal gait characterized by foot supination and lateral border walking[24] as well as compensatory hyperextension at the hallucal interphalangeal joint. This condition is referred to as hallux rigidus, a progressive degenerative joint disease secondary to biomechanical disturbance or arthritic pathologic abnormality that ultimately results in ankylosis of the joint. Hallux rigidus can present insidiously or posttraumatically with pain, stiffness, and a dorsal bunion localized at the first MTP joint. Symptoms are associated with activities that require extension of the first MTP, such as squatting, stooping, or high-heeled shoe wear.[26]

Deformities of the lesser digits are classically referred to as hammer toes, claw toes, and mallet toes (**Fig. 4**). These conditions may be congenital, acquired, or a component of other disorders. Like HVD, lesser toe deformities may be asymptomatic or present with varying degrees of pain secondary to bursitis, calluses, contracture, or shifts in pressure. Trauma such as fractures should be ruled out especially in an acute presentation of pain. Arthritic conditions may manifest with symptoms affecting the lesser digit joints, especially rheumatoid, and should be considered. A full evaluation includes gait assessment, ROM testing for flexibility, and palpation. Applying direct dorsal and plantar stress to the MTP joints will assess for instability often associated with

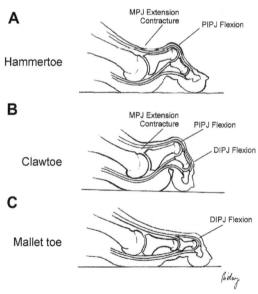

Fig. 4. Three common digital deformities. In general, they can be described as the combination of joint contractures at the digital segments: (A) hammer toes have flexion at the proximal interphalangeal joint (PIPJ) with extension at the metatarsophalangeal joint (MPJ) with a neutral or hyperextended distal interphalangeal joint (DIPJ), (B) claw toes have flexion at both the PIPJ and the DIPJ combined with extension at the MPJ, (C) mallet toes have flexion at the DIPJ. (*From* Thomas JL, Blitch EL, Chaney DM, et al. Diagnosis and treatment of forefoot disorders. Section 1: digital deformities. J Foot Ankle Surg 2009;48(2):230–8; with permission.)

claw toes.[13] Radiographs can be used to gauge severity and degeneration and monitor progression of all digital deformities.[25] PRICERM is the first-line treatment.

VASCULAR FUNCTION

Pulses are assessed by using the pads of the index and middle fingers to apply the lightest possible pressure to avoid compressing the vessels. The posterior tibial artery pulse can be palpated in the tarsal canal in the groove between the medial malleolus and the Achilles tendon.[27] It is best felt when the foot is completely relaxed. The anterior tibial artery is renamed the dorsalis pedis artery (DPA) after it crosses the ankle. Only 3% of patients have a congenitally absent DPA.[29] The DPA is found along the dorsum of the foot lateral to the extensor hallucis longus tendon and medial to the extensor digitorum longus tendon. Starting at the navicular tuberosity, gently palpating across an arc over the dorsum of the foot toward the lateral malleolus in a posterior-lateral direction can help detect the pulse. Plantarflexion of the foot is avoided because this decreases sensitivity of palpation.[27]

Peripheral Vascular Disease

Diminished or absent pulses, temperature changes, bluish nail beds, and shiny or atrophied skin are significant signs of peripheral artery disease (PAD). Subtle changes in temperature can be appreciated by moving the dorsal surface of the hand proximally from the toes.[30] PAD affects 10% of the population and is a marker for general artherosclerotic disease. Intermittent claudication—pain reproduced by exercise and relieved by rest—is the classical presentation of PAD seen in 30% to 40% of all cases. Foot claudication can result from occlusion of the tibial or peroneal artery, although this is less common than proximal (eg, popliteal) artery stenosis.[31] The diagnosis of PAD may be confounded by comorbidities that present with similar pain. It may be confused with neurogenic claudication because of spinal stenosis. A key distinction between vascular and neurogenic claudication is forward bending—this enlarges the spinal canal and improves the symptoms of neurogenic but not vascular pain.[28] In diabetics, PAD increases both morbidity and mortality. It rarely leads to ulcerations directly, but once ulceration develops, it will heal poorly because of decreased perfusion. Subsequent infections are difficult to eradicate because of inadequate oxygenation and antibiotic delivery.[12]

Swelling

Fluid extravasation presenting as swelling is common following traumatic and inflammatory tissue disturbance. Swelling may be extensive, affecting the entire lower extremity or localized at a joint. It is frequently accompanied by rubor, pain, and limited ROM. Most cases of unilateral swelling result from acute inflammatory processes.[18] Cellulitis, deep vein thrombosis, compartment syndrome, and acute Charcot foot (CN) may all present with diffuse lower extremity swelling. Bilateral swelling is common in patients with venous insufficiency, which is frequently accompanied by stasis dermatitis, pain, blisters, and ulceration. Pulmonary hypertension and early heart failure are other possible causes of bilateral edema seen frequently in older individuals.[32]

The ankle and first MTP joints are the most common sites of swelling. Septic effusions should remain on the differential of any acute monoarticular inflammation until definitively ruled out.[18] In the ankle, fluid may pool around both malleoli and the dorsal foot in response to traumatic damage, such as sprains, or systemic conditions, such as gout or rheumatoid arthritis.[24] Swelling associated with HVD may be confused with gouty inflammation because both affect the first MTP joint. Gout is common in older men with a positive family history or prior attack and does not have the characteristic valgus deviation of HVD unless the conditions are superimposed. It is aggravated by trauma, surgery, alcohol, dietary factors, or dehydration.[18] Gout and pseudogout are diagnosed by the presence of crystals in the synovial fluid obtained by joint aspiration. Arthrocentesis is often necessary for assessment of other conditions as well. Normal synovial fluid is clear with a slight yellow tinge. Aspirated fluid that looks purulent or blood-tinged requires urgent attention. The characteristic appearance of purulent fluid is due to an increased white blood cell count (greater than 50,000/mm³) and is usually a response to infection. Blood-tinged synovial fluid is referred to as hemarthrosis. A traumatic tap or history of anticoagulant use or hemophilia may explain the presence of blood.[28] Hemarthrosis may also be suggestive of an intra-articular fracture or a ligament tear. If fat droplets are seen on microscopic analysis, joint fracture is even more likely. Aspirated fluid should be sent for analysis that includes a total leukocyte count with differential, Gram stain, cultures and special stains, sensitivities, glucose, and crystal examination.[18] In cases of septic arthritis, antibiotics can be adjusted or discontinued after culture results are available.

Arthrocentesis is simple to perform in an office setting. Consent and proper sterile technique should not be forgotten. A 25-gauge needle is used for small joints. The ankle is aspirated from an anteromedial approach by palpating the depression between the medial malleolus and anterior tibial tendon. The needle is inserted to a depth of 1 to 3 cm, aiming toward the middle of the ankle joint. Aspiration of the first MTP joint is done using a medial approach to help avoid tendons and neurovasculature. With the joint in 15° of flexion, the needle is inserted straight in at the depression between the 2 bones. Aspiration may be used therapeutically to decompress any joint in the absence of relative contraindications, such as clotting disorders and infection of the surrounding tissue.[18]

NEUROLOGIC ASSESSMENT

Proprioception should be universally assessed with the Romberg test as a part of general evaluation—especially in patients with prior ankle injuries or peripheral neuropathies (PN). Starting with the unaffected side, patients should stand on one foot for at least 5 seconds with their eyes open and then with eyes closed.[1] Mechanoreceptors located in ligaments provide most of the proprioceptive information. Any damage will compromise normal function, leading to chronic ankle issues, such as instability, further injuries, and falls in the elderly.[33] Inability to hold the position with eyes closed for the appropriate time is an indication for rehabilitation.

Neuropathies

PN is commonly seen in a primary care setting. There is a long list of broadly grouped causes including genetic disorders, substance toxicity, inflammatory diseases, vitamin deficiencies, and traumatic injury. Diabetic PN is by far the most likely cause in America; a classic history may include symmetric weakness in toes and distal sensory loss in a stocking and glove distribution. The sensory or motor arc of the deep tendon reflexes can be diminished or completely absent in any PN.[28] Reflexes are tested by stretching the tendon with a brisk tap of a reflex hammer and observing the immediate muscle contraction. Reflexes are best tested in a sitting position with the patient relaxed and not thinking about the procedure. Multiple samples of the reflex should be taken to assess reactivity. Normal reflexes confirm appropriate cutaneous and motor innervation as well as normal cortical input into the tested spinal nerve segment.[34] There is also normal variation in deep tendon reflexes and diminished or increased reflexes without other clinical findings are usually not pathologic.

Constant vigilance is required when caring for diabetic patients and physicians should be current on all appropriate screening techniques.[7] Unfortunately, patient education on foot care does not produce clinically relevant reduction in complications.[35] The lifetime risk of developing foot ulcers is as high as 25% in diabetics and PN is the universal predisposing factor.[7] In addition to neuropathy, vascular disease is a factor in up to 45% of diabetic ulcerations.[12] Approximately 1% of diabetics will develop an inflammatory neuropathic arthropathy known as Charcot Neuroarthropathy (CN) due to a lack of protective sensation, which leads to damage and degeneration of weight-bearing joints.[36] A history of injury is unreliable because more than half of the patients have decreased or absent pain perception. There is a significantly increased risk of severe traumas or infections that may go unnoticed for prolonged periods.[14] The acute clinical presentation of CN usually includes a swollen, erythematous lower extremity with bounding pedal pulses and a temperature differential.[36] The associated hyperemia increases bone reabsorption. Gross deformities may be subtle in early stages.[12] Chronic CN presentation includes the hallmark midfoot structural collapse referred to as a rocker bottom foot (**Fig. 5**).[36] CN is limb threatening and requires prompt treatment to reduce the swelling. Acute CN is often misdiagnosed with other conditions common in diabetics, such as cellulitis, deep vein thrombosis, or osteomyelitis. Plain films are appropriate initial studies but magnetic resonance imaging (MRI) is the most accurate. Rubor associated with CN is dependent and will resolve within 10 minutes of foot elevation but erythema associated with infection will not.[37]

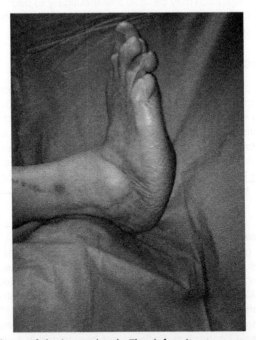

Fig. 5. CN with collapse of the internal arch. The deformity can occur abruptly and usually without any relevant preceding trauma. Late-stage CN often presents a rocker-bottom deformity. (*From* Hartemann-Heurtier A, Van GH, Grimaldi A. The Charcot foot. Lancet 2002;360(9347):1776–9.)

Nerve Entrapment Syndromes

PN from nonsystemic causes is usually due to stretching, entrapment, or compression of nerves and tends to be unilateral (**Table 2**).[38] The diagnosis is clinical.[39,40] Classic symptoms of include pain worsened by weight-bearing, deep burning, paresthesias, and numbness in the nerve's distribution distal to the site of damage. Weakness and atrophy of intrinsic muscles of the foot are very late findings. Stretching- or tension-related nerve disorders occur from acute ankle sprains or inappropriate foot mechanics.[38,40] External pressures from improper footwear and space-occupying masses, such as scar tissue, bone spurs, varicose veins, or focal swelling, are the usual culprits responsible for nerve compression or entrapment.[38]

Tinel sign is a sensitive but not specific finding elicited by gentle percussion over the nerve path useful for diagnosing neuropathies.[41] A positive sign involves tingling as well as pins and needles in the nerve distribution (**Fig. 6**).[24] In the case of tarsal tunnel syndrome, a positive test is 88% to 93% predictive of excellent postsurgical outcomes.[41] However, there is significant inter- and intra-examiner variability in technique and the amount of force applied. The "single finger technique"—5 strikes using only the middle finger of the dominant hand—produces relatively minimal intragroup variability (**Fig. 7**).[42] The triple compression stress test is most diagnostic with a sensitivity and specificity of 85.9% and 100%, respectively.[43] A compressive force held for 30 seconds on the posterior tibial nerve with the foot in plantarflexion and inversion should elicit pain and numbness if the test is positive (**Fig. 8**).

Baxter neuropathy, entrapment of the motor branch of the lateral plantar nerve, is responsible for 20% of chronic heel pain but is frequently overlooked.[38] Diagnosis is based on the pathognomonic MRI finding of selective fatty atrophy of the abductor digiti minimi. Imaging studies are not required for other PNs but can be used to determine cause or rule out other pathologic abnormalities if surgery is planned.[44] MRI is very accurate[39,45] but diagnostic ultrasound is gaining popularity because of lower costs.[46] Electrodiagnostic studies have high false positive and negative rates and are not diagnostically superior to provocative tests.[43]

PN that presents in late childhood or early adulthood is suspicious for congenital causes. Charcot-Marie-Tooth disease is one of the most common hereditary nervous system conditions. It is heterogeneous with variable inheritance. It can be recessive so a negative family history does not exclude the diagnosis. Charcot-Marie-Tooth presents with muscle weakness, foot deformity (foot drop, high arches, hammer toes), or sensory loss.[47] Other causes of PNs should be excluded. Definitive diagnosis is made by nerve biopsy or genetic testing.[48]

PALPATION OF STRUCTURES

Most patients with foot and ankle complaints present with regional pain or discomfort. Reproduction of symptoms through provocation is necessary to make a diagnosis. The foot has a minimum of 26 key bones in addition to at least 2 sesamoids, many ligaments stabilizing the joints, fascia, as well as intrinsic and extrinsic musculature.[28] Pain, swelling, and dysfunction can originate from disruption of any of these components. Knowledge of anatomy is crucial. Many disorders can be noticed clinically by pairing relevant historical findings with localization of a specific point of tenderness (**Fig. 9**). Palpation of skin and subcutaneous tissues is performed by applying varying degrees of pressure with finger pads. Deeper structures require firm pressure and may be better appreciated when the foot is manipulated or actively moved. Deformity, asymmetry, crepitus, tenderness, elasticity, and texture of the palpated structures should be noted. When performing a complete assessment, palpation should be

Table 2
Nerve impingement syndromes in the foot

	Location of Compression	External Landmarks	Presentation	Diagnostic Tests (Sensitivity/Specificity)
Tarsal tunnel syndrome Nerve: tibial or its divisional branches	Beneath flexor retinaculum on medial aspect of ankle	Posterior to medial malleolus; medial to talus and calcaneus	*Onset:* Insidious *Symptoms:* Pain directly over the tarsal tunnel; radiation to longitudinal arch, plantar foot and heel. Can be worse at night *Aggravated by:* Standing, walking	• Tinels sign • Triple compression stress test: (85.9%/100%) • MRI: (83%)
Baxter's neuropathy Nerve: inferior calcaneal	Between inferior margin of abductor hallucis (AbH) and quadratus plantae	Anterior to medial calcaneus; almost in line with medial malleolus	*Onset:* Insidious *Symptoms:* Chronic heel pain; can be confused with or accompanied by plantar fasciitis; radiation to inferomedial heel and medial ankle. Can be worse in the morning	• MRI: selective fatty atrophy of abductor digiti minimi is a unique finding
Jogger's foot Nerve: medial plantar	Passage between AbH and the knot of Henry	Plantar, one thumb breadth distal to navicular tuberosity	*Onset:* Immediately after running *Symptoms:* Burning heel and medial arch pain; sensory disturbance over plantar surface behind first and second toes	• Tinel sign • Passive foot eversion • MRI: denervation changes in muscles supplied

Morton's neuroma Nerve: interdigital branches of medial plantar	Fibrosis due to chronic impingement against distal edge of plantar intermetatarsal ligament	Plantar forefoot over third and fourth metatarsals and in third web space	*Onset:* Usually insidious *Symptoms:* Paroxysmal pain in plantar foot, toes, and dorsal web space; radiates from metatarsal heads to third and fourth toes; altered sensation in less than half *Aggravated by:* All shoes, high heels	• Tinel sign: (62%) • Web space tenderness (95%) • Squeeze test: (88%) • MRI: (87%/100%)
Anterior tarsal tunnel syndrome Nerve: deep peroneal	Under superior edge of inferior retinaculum	Level of talonavicular joint, lateral to the drosalis pedis artery	*Onset:* Acute or chronic if caused by tight fitting shoes *Symptoms:* Pain of dorsomedial midfoot; minimal weakness of extensor hallucis brevis (EHB); sensory disturbance in first webspace. Worse at night or at rest	• Tinel sign • Ultrasound >>MRI

Data from Refs.[10,16–19,24]

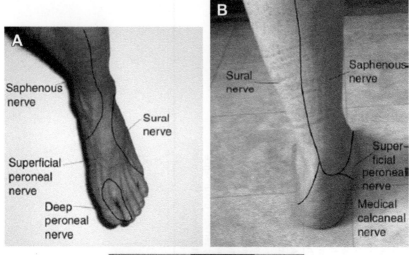

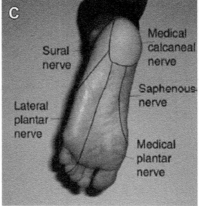

Fig. 6. Typical sensory innervation of the foot and ankle. (*A*) Superior view (*B*) Posterior view and (*C*) Inferior view. (*From* Young CC, Niedfeldt MW, Morris GA, et al. Clinical examination of the foot and ankle. Prim Care 2005;32(1):105–32; with permission.)

done systematically starting proximally above the ankle and moving distally through the hindfoot, midfoot, and forefoot. Areas of reported pain should be assessed last to avoid patient discomfort.

Ottawa Foot and Ankle Rules

In the setting of any suspected foot or ankle injury, patients should be evaluated following the Ottawa Ankle Rules (OAR) to exclude fractures and avoid unnecessary radiography (**Fig. 10**). To apply the rules correctly, the physician should palpate the entire distal 6 cm of the fibula and tibia; remember the importance of medial malleolar tenderness; palpate the entirety of the navicular, with special attention to the relatively avascular nickel-sized area at the central region of the proximal dorsal surface termed the "N" spot; palpate the fifth metatarsal focusing on the base; note verbal and nonverbal pain responses; observe the patient ambulate for at least 4 steps. Tenderness at these locations is an indication for radiographs. Standard imaging includes

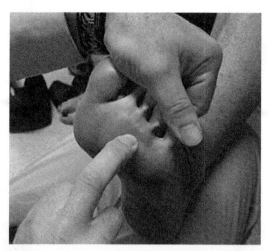

Fig. 7. Demonstration of the single finger percussion technique. (*From* Owens R, Gougoulias N, Guthrie H, et al. Morton's neuroma: clinical testing and imaging in 76 feet, compared to a control group. Foot Ankle Surg 2011;17(3):197–200; with permission.)

anterior to posterior, lateral, and ankle mortise views. There are 11 important sites to assess when evaluating patients for low-energy fractures (**Fig. 11**).[49]

These rules have been validated in multiple clinical settings with varying prevalence of fractures, in adult patients, and in children greater than 5 years of age.[50] If a patient has negative findings following the OAR, there is less than a 2% chance that this is a false negative.[51] Limited knowledge of OAR may preclude implementation in practice—in a study, 99.2% of providers were aware of the rules but only 30.9% were able to recall all the components correctly. In patients with repeat injuries, chronic or worsening symptoms, or a difficult clinical assessment, radiographs should be obtained regardless of the rules.[52] Specificity of palpation is limited by extensive soft tissue edema.[24] If a grossly swollen ankle prevents proper palpation of bony structures, radiographs should be obtained.[52]

Overuse Injuries

Running is the common denominator in many foot and ankle injuries. Sudden increases in training volume or a history of prior injuries are major risk factors for all running-based injuries. Variables such as gait, incline, pace, interval training, and

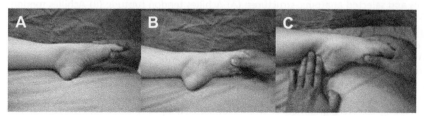

Fig. 8. The triple compression stress test involves 3 steps: (*A*) place ankle in plantar flexion, (*B*) invert the heel and foot, and (*C*) compress the tibial nerve where it runs posterior to the medial malleolus. (*From* Abouelela AA, Zohiery AK. The triple compression stress test for diagnosis of tarsal tunnel syndrome. Foot (Edinb) 2012;22(3):146–9. Elsevier Ltd; with permission.)

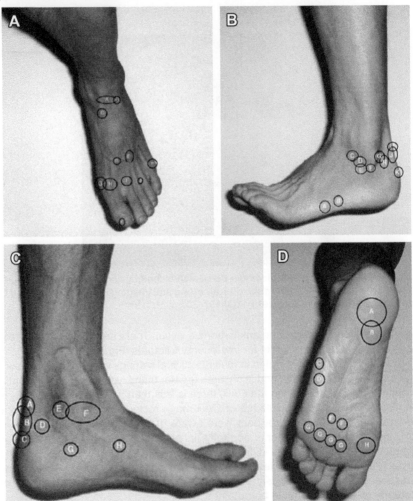

Fig. 9. Important palpation landmarks. (*B*) Lateral foot and ankle—typical locations of injury symptoms and selected anatomic structures: (A) Jones fracture; (B) avulsion fracture of the fifth metatarsal; (C) anterior ankle impingement; (D) anterior talofibular ligament; (E) sinus tarsi; (F) calcaneofibular ligament; (G) posterior ankle impingement; (H) retrocalcaneal bursitis; (I) Achilles tendon rupture; (J) Achilles tendonitis; (K) calcaneal apophysitis (Sever condition) and "pump bump." (*C*) Medial foot and ankle—typical locations of injury symptoms and selected anatomic structures: (A) Achilles tendon rupture; (B) Achilles tendonitis; (C) calcaneal apophysitis (Sever condition) and "pump bump"; (D) retrocalcaneal bursitis; (E) tarsal tunnel syndrome; (F) medial ankle sprain; (G) entrapment site of first branch of lateral plantar nerve; (H) master knot of Henry, entrapment site of medial plantar nerve. (*A*) Dorsal foot and ankle—typical locations of injury symptoms and selected anatomic structures: (A) anterior ankle impingement; (B) osteochondritis dissecans of the lateral talar dome; (C) the N spot—NSF; (D) Lisfranc sprain; (E) anterior tarsal tunnel syndrome; (F) bunionette; (G) bunion; (H) hallux rigidus; (I) avascular necrosis of second metatarsal head (Freiberg infarction); (J) interdigital neuroma (Morton neuroma); (K) paronychia. (*D*) Plantar foot—typical locations of injury symptoms and selected anatomic structures: (A) plantar fat pad; (B) plantar fasciitis; (C) avulsion fracture of the fifth metatarsal; (D) Jones fracture; (E) stress fracture of the third metatarsal; (F) stress fracture of the second metatarsal; (G) metatarsalgia; (H) sesamoiditis. (*From* Young CC, Niedfeldt MW, Morris GA, et al. Clinical examination of the foot and ankle. Prim Care 2005;32(1):105–32; with permission.)

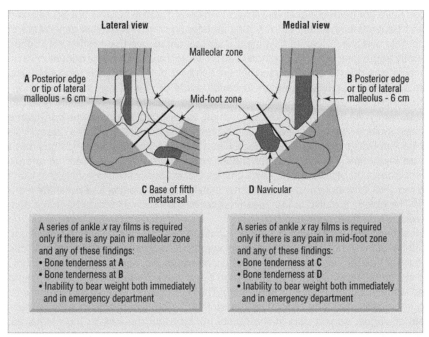

Fig. 10. Ottowa ankle rules. (*From* Bachmann LM, Kolb E, Koller MT, et al. Accuracy of Ottawa ankle rules to exclude fractures of the ankle and mid-foot: systematic review. BMJ 2003;326(7386):417; with permission.)

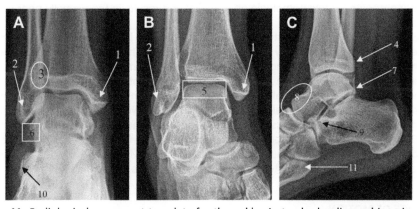

Fig. 11. Radiological assessment template for the ankle. A standard radiographic series of the ankle has a minimum of 3 views including an anterior-posterior view (*A*), a mortise view (*B*), and a lateral view (*C*). There are 11 target sites that represent vulnerable areas where fractures occur including the medial (1) and lateral (2) malleoli, anterior tibial tubercle (3) and posterior tibial malleolus (4), talar dome (5), lateral talar process (6), tubercles of the posterior talus process (7), dorsal to the talonavicular joint (8), anterior calcaneus process (9), calcaneal insertion of the extensor digitorum brevis (10), and the base of the fifth metatarsal bone (11). (*From* Yu JS, Cody ME. A template approach for detecting fractures in adults sustaining low-energy ankle trauma. Emerg Radiol 2009;16(4):309–18; with permission.)

shoes have not been conclusively linked to injuries.[53] Ankle sprains are acute and the most frequent injury sustained by young athletes, but most injuries in general are due to chronic overuse.[8] Despite a typically insidious onset, overuse injuries may become abruptly aggravated and misdiagnosed as an acute trauma. Damage occurs from relative overload due to an increased tissue demand but inadequate recovery. Single events are not significant enough to cause acute problems but the culmination of microscopic damage from repetitive application of force will eventually result in a serious injury. All tissue types are susceptible to this mechanism; some common examples include navicular, calcaneal, or metatarsal stress fractures, apophysitis, plantar fasciitis, and Achilles tendinopathies.[28] Underlying medical conditions may increase injury risk. Female patients should be evaluated for "the Triad" of anorexia, amenorrhea, and osteoporosis. This constellation is usually seen in young, thin women and requires intervention to prevent other significant morbidities and potential mortality.[28] The elderly are also at increased risk for injuries such as stress fractures due to osteopenia or osteoporosis.[54]

Most overuse injuries lead to chronic localized pain.[55] Patients will often attempt to continue activity but this only leads to symptom progression: the pain will occur earlier, last longer, and eventually lead to complications, such as arthritis, nonunion, and structural deformity.[56] A very common injury that is frequently missed or mismanaged is the navicular stress fracture (NSF). The navicular is the point of maximal stress and impingement during repetitive foot strikes.[57] NSF symptoms include a gradual onset of vague, aching pain in the dorsal midfoot that radiates to the medial arch. Edema and ecchymosis are usually absent. Patients will experience increased pain with passive eversion, active inversion, toe hopping, and toe standing. Tenderness localized to the "N" spot is present in 81% of patients and is an indication for imaging according to the OAR. However, plain films are only sensitive in 33% of acute cases and a follow-up foot MRI is appropriate.[58] Treatment involves non-weight-bearing cast immobilization for 6 to 8 weeks. Many physicians default to PRICEMR, which is inappropriate for this pathologic abnormality and results in the dismally poor cure rate of 26%.[55]

Similar to NSF, calcaneal stress fractures are overuse injuries that present shortly after an increase in frequency or intensity of activity.[59] They are classically descried in new military recruits or long distance runners.[54] The most common site of injury is immediately inferior to the posterior facet of the subtalar joint and presents as tenderness of the lateral wall of the calcaneus.[59] Pain elicited by the calcaneal compression test—compression of the heel in a transverse plane by both palms (**Fig. 12**)—is highly suspicious.[59] Vibration applied to the calcaneus using either a 128-cps tuning fork or ultrasound can cause discomfort.[24] Onset of symptoms precedes radiographic findings but 3-phase bone scans or MRIs are nearly 100% sensitive as early as 1 to 2 days after injury.[53] Treatment is the same as NSF.

RANGE OF MOTION
Terminology

To evaluate and understand disorders of the foot and ankle, an understanding of the planes of motion and positions of the foot are essential to assess these disorders and effectively communicate pertinent findings when referring to health providers.

The upper surface of the foot is the dorsum of the foot and the bottom or weight-bearing surface is the plantar aspect. The medial side of the foot is the side closest to the midline. The lateral side is furthest away from the midline. Medial and lateral may also be described as the tibial and fibular borders, respectively. There are 3 basic

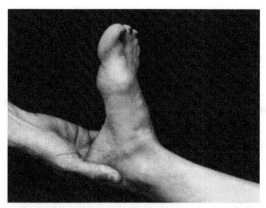

Fig. 12. Calcaneal compression test. (*From* DiGiovanni, BF, Dawson, LK, Baumhauer, JF. Plantar Heel Pain. In: Coughlin, MJ, Saltzman, CL, Anderson, RB, editors. Mann's Surgery of the Foot and Ankle. 9th edition. Philadelphia, PA: Elsevier; 2014. p. 685–701; with permission.)

planes of motion involving the foot and ankle complex. There are sagittal, frontal, and transverse planes of motion. Dorsiflexion and plantarflexion are considered sagittal motions. A fixed position would be described as either plantarflexed or dorsiflexed. Inversion and eversion occur along frontal plane. Inversion occurs when the foot is rotated toward the midline; eversion is rotation of the foot away from the midline. The foot when it is in a fixed position would be described as being in varus; the foot fixed in an everted position would be in valgus. Transverse motion is described as adduction and abduction. Motion toward the midline is adduction; motion away from the midline is abduction. Fixed position in the transverse plane is adduction and abduction. Supination and pronation, while often used to describe foot patterns, more specifically represents composite motion in all 3 planes. Supination is adduction, inversion, and plantarflexion of the foot. Pronation involves abduction, eversion, and dorsiflexion of the foot.

Ligament and articular geometry are the primary determinants of available ROM, but all structural components play a vital role in normal function.[60] Resisted ROM is often used clinically to gauge muscle strength; the physician exerts a force against the muscle being tested using personal strength as a gauge for normality while the lower extremity is stabilized to avoid substitution by proximal muscles.[28] Strength is best evaluated in functional weight-bearing positions and during ambulation if possible—patients should walk on heels, toes, as well as lateral and medial borders of the foot.[1] Passive ROM is used for assessing the integrity of joints and their supporting structures. Normal joints should move smoothly and the end point should be firm.[61] Pain, laxity, catching, locking, or inappropriate end point quality are pathologic. Passive ROM requires patient cooperation; the procedure should be explained and the patient asked to allow movement without active resistance.[62] The hindfoot is capable of complex triplanar motion through action at the ankle and subtalar joints. The lateral ligament complex and the medial deltoid ligament play a large role in stabilizing the hindfoot and preventing excessive translation.[8] The lateral ligament complex includes the anterior talofibular ligament, the calcaneofibular ligament, and the posterior talofibular ligament and damage to these structures results in pathologic joint movement. The ankle or "mortise" is a synovial hinge joint, involving the articulation between the tibia, fibula, and talus. This joint is responsible for sagittal movement and the average patient is capable of 20° dorsiflexion and up to 50° of plantarflexion.[28] Bone spurs or accessory bones such as the os trigonum can cause painful impingement syndromes that limit ROM at the ankle. Symptoms can be reproduced by sharp dorsiflexion or plantarflexion resulting in pain at the anterior or posterior joint line, respectively.[24] The subtalar joint is a synovial, bicondylar compound joint that consists of the anterior, middle, and posterior articulation surfaces between the talus and the calcaneus. There is great variability in subtalar motion, but the average individual should have an inversion range of 5° to 40° and an eversion range of 5° to 20°. Ankle ROM should be assessed with the knee flexed and then extended. The hindfoot should be in a neutral position and the forefoot locked in inversion. Although one hand stabilizes the heel, the other should use the midfoot as a lever to maximally dorsiflex and plantarflex the joint. In the same position, subtalar ROM can be tested by slowly turning the heel in and out.[28] Most of the remaining articulations are relatively static and their ROM is not routinely assessed. The individual bones of the midfoot, for example, are only capable of minimal independent motion because of numerous ligaments that bind the structures together; this is functionally crucial for shock absorption during ambulation.[63]

GAIT ASSESSMENT

Patients rarely present with gait disturbance as a chief complaint but difficulty walking is a common secondary problem.[64] Gait assessment is arguably the most important aspect in the clinical evaluation of FAD. Normal gait requires the coordination between the nervous and musculoskeletal systems and relies heavily on intact sensory information from the visual, vestibular, and proprioceptive systems. There are many ways to evaluate gait using sophisticated equipment; however, visual observation is quick and can give much information in a cost-effective manner.[1] Ambulation should be systematically assessed from the front, side, and back. The stance phase takes up about 60% of the gait cycle and the swing phase takes up the remaining 40%. The overall pattern of body movement should be evaluated first for posture, symmetry, fluidity, temporal parameters, cadence, stance, and step length.[65] Next, the motion at individual joints should be observed from the feet upward to help differentiate a focal problem in the lower extremity from a generalized movement disorder.[64] Calcaneal motion can be monitored by marking the midline of the rear foot and watching the movement through the entire gait cycle.[1] Increasing the pace may bring out subtle disorders. Antalgic gait can be caused by any painful condition in the lower extremity, such as arthritis, ankle sprains, and stress fractures of the foot. The characteristic limp is a result of decreased time in the stance phase of the affected limb in an attempt to minimize pain with weight-bearing and can be recognized as a decrease in step length of the uninjured side and overall decrease in velocity.[64] The ability to ambulate for at least 4 steps regardless of gait is a criterion in the OAR.

Gait and Falls in the Elderly

There are many causes and patterns for gait disturbances, especially in the elderly population. Up to 15% of patients older than 64 years and more than 40% of patients over 85 years have a gait abnormality. Balance and gait impairment nearly double the risk for falling, which can result in serious soft tissue injuries and fractures.[64] Other risk factors, such as the use of sedatives, environmental hazards, and excessive medication, should be modified.[28] Not all abnormal gaits are concerning. Nonpathologic age-related changes include shorter and broader-based steps, decreased velocity, and decreased step length.[65] Pathologic movement disorders in the elderly are most commonly due to cerebral infarcts, arthritic pain, spinal spondylopathy, Parkinson disease, and cerebellar degeneration.[64]

Sensory ataxia is a gait pattern that results from disruption of afferent pathways in the visual, vestibular, or proprioceptive systems. The patient loses awareness of limb position but muscle strength remains intact. The most common cause in America is likely diabetes-related polyneuropathy with visual disturbances. This gait is characterized by a wide stance and a forceful slap on contact with the floor to increase sensory feedback. Patients are often vigilantly watching the ground during ambulation and will have dramatic instability in the darkness or when asked to perform the Romberg test. The slap associated with sensory ataxia may be confused with the slapping of foot drop from deficits in strength of the ankle dorsiflexors, but other clinical findings easily distinguish the 2 patterns. There are numerous causes for foot drop including acquired or hereditary peripheral neuropathies, peroneal nerve injuries, radiculopathy at L4, or loss of motion at the ankle.[64] A steppage gait with excessive hip and knee flexion is used to help the toes clear the ground during the swing phase.[24] Toes will make contact with the ground before heel strike, producing the characteristic slap.

Special Consideration in High-Energy Falls

Fall-related injuries can be intentional, such as a suicide attempt, accidental, such as falling off the roof, or simply poor judgment, such as a teenager jumping out of a window.[28] Falls are emergencies because of the high potential for soft tissue injuries and fractures of the pelvis, thoracolumbar spine, and skull base.[66] The physical examination should include assessment of the skin for open wounds, neurovascular integrity, and a thorough musculoskeletal evaluation.[67] Feet-first impact is the most common falling mechanism resulting in calcaneal fractures.[67] Patients present with varying degrees of heel tenderness, swelling, ecchymosis, and loss of heel contour but still may be able to bear weight.[68] Many other fracture sites and patterns exist.

SUMMARY

Most FAD can be diagnosed after a proper clinical examination and managed in a primary care setting. It is important to assess the patient as a whole because age, gender, athletic involvement, and pre-existing medical conditions determine which common conditions are common in a given patient population. A broad differential should include disorders of bones, joints, muscles, neurovasculature, and surrounding soft tissue structures. Physical examination should localize the area of maximal tenderness and assess the effect of the problem on ROM, strength, and gait. Symptom reproduction is often fundamental to making a diagnosis. Imaging should be used only when the potential findings are likely to change the diagnosis or management to limit unnecessary expense and radiation.

REFERENCES

1. Giallonardo LM. Clinical evaluation of foot and ankle dysfunction. Phys Ther 1988;68(12):1850–6.
2. Jordan K, Kadam U, Hayward R, et al. Annual consultation prevalence of regional musculoskeletal problems in primary care: an observational study. BMC Musculoskelet Disord 2010;11:144–54.
3. Parsons S, Breen A, Foster NE, et al. Prevalence and comparative troublesomeness by age of musculoskeletal pain in different body locations. Fam Pract 2007;24(4):308–16.
4. Mølgaard C, Lundbye-Christensen S, Simonsen O. High prevalence of foot problems in the Danish population: a survey of causes and associations. Foot (Edinb) 2010;20(1):7–11.

5. Kelly JC, Groarke PJ, Flanagan E, et al. Foot and ankle surgery–the Achilles heel of medical students and doctors. Foot (Edinb) 2011;21(3):109–13 Elsevier Ltd.

6. Woolf AD, Akesson K. Primer: history and examination in the assessment of musculoskeletal problems. Nat Clin Pract Rheumatol 2008;4(1):26–33.

7. Boulton AJ, Armstrong DG, Albert SF, et al. Comprehensive foot examination and risk assessment: a report of the task force of the foot care interest group of the American Diabetes Association, with endorsement by the American Association of Clinical Endocrinologists. Diabetes Care 2008;31(8):1679–85.

8. Lynch SA. Assessment of the injured ankle in the athlete. J Athl Train 2002;37(4):406–12.

9. Hewitt S, Yates B, Williamson D. A prospective audit of referral patterns to a dedicated foot and ankle surgical service. Foot (Edinb) 2011;21(4):166–71 Elsevier Ltd.

10. Simpson MR, Howard TM. Tendinopathies of the foot and ankle. Am Fam Physician 2009;80(10):1107–14.

11. Butterworth PA, Landorf KB, Smith SE, et al. The association between body mass index and musculoskeletal foot disorders: a systematic review. Obes Rev 2012;13(7):630–42.

12. Frykberg RG, Zgonis T, Armstrong DG, et al. Diabetic foot disorders. A clinical practice guideline (2006 revision). J Foot Ankle Surg 2006;45(Suppl 5):S1–66.

13. Thomas JL, Blitch EL, Chaney DM, et al. Diagnosis and treatment of forefoot disorders. Section 1: digital deformities. J Foot Ankle Surg 2009;48(2):230–8.

14. Anakwenze O, Milby A, Gans I, et al. Foot and ankle infections: diagnosis and management. J Am Acad Orthop Surg 2012;20:684–93.

15. Liu C, Bayer A, Cosgrove SE, et al. Clinical practice guidelines by the Infectious Diseases Society of America for the treatment of methicillin-resistant Staphylococcus aureus infections in adults and children. Clin Infect Dis 2011;52(3):e18–55.

16. Perlman MH, Patzakis MJ, Kumar PJ, et al. The incidence of joint involvement with adjacent osteomyelitis in pediatric patients. J Pediatr Orthop 2000;20(1):40–3.

17. Perron AD, Brady WJ, Miller MD. Orthopedic pitfalls in the ED: osteomyelitis. Am J Emerg Med 2003;21(1):61–7.

18. Mackie JW. Joint aspiration: arthrocentesis. Can Fam Physician 1987;33(10):2057–62.

19. Saavedra-Lozano J, Mejías A, Ahmad N, et al. Changing trends in acute osteomyelitis in children: impact of methicillin-resistant Staphylococcus aureus infections. J Pediatr Orthop 2008;28(5):569–75.

20. Harris EJ, Vanore JV, Thomas JL, et al. Diagnosis and treatment of pediatric flatfoot. J Foot Ankle Surg 2004;43(6):341–73.

21. Nix S, Smith M, Vicenzino B. Prevalence of hallux valgus in the general population: a systematic review and meta-analysis. J Foot Ankle Res 2010;3:21–9.

22. Mosca VS. Flexible flatfoot in children and adolescents. J Child Orthop 2010;4(2):107–21.

23. Sass P, Hassan G. Lower extremity abnormalities in children. Am Fam Physician 2003;68(3):461–8.

24. Young CC, Niedfeldt MW, Morris GA, et al. Clinical examination of the foot and ankle. Prim Care 2005;32(1):105–32.

25. Vanore JV, Christensen JC, Kravitz SR, et al. Diagnosis and treatment of first metatarsophalangeal joint disorders. Section 1: Hallux valgus. J Foot Ankle Surg 2003;42(3):112–23.

26. Nix SE, Vicenzino BT, Collins NJ, et al. Gait parameters associated with hallux valgus: a systematic review. J Foot Ankle Res 2013;6(1):9.
27. Hobson J, Bicknell C, Cheshire N. Dorsalis pedis arterial pulse: palpation using a bony landmark. Postgrad Med J 2003;79(932):363.
28. Bernstein J, editor. Musculoskeletal medicine. 1st edition. Rosemont (IL): American Academy of Orthopaedic Surgeons; 2003.
29. Robertson GS, Ristic CD, Bullen BR. The incidence of congenitally absent foot pulses. Ann R Coll Surg Engl 1990;72(2):99–100.
30. Khan NA, Rahim SA, Anand SS, et al. Does the clinical examination predict lower extremity peripheral arterial disease? JAMA 2006;295(5):536–46.
31. Dhaliwal G, Mukherjee D. Peripheral arterial disease: epidemiology, natural history, diagnosis and treatment. Int J Angiol 2007;16(2):36–44.
32. Ely JW, Osheroff JA, Chambliss ML, et al. Approach to leg edema of unclear etiology. J Am Board Fam Med 2006;19(2):148–60.
33. Tiemstra JD. Update on acute ankle sprains. Am Fam Physician 2012;85(12): 1170–6.
34. Walker H. Deep tendon reflexes. In: HK W, Hall W, Hurst J, editors. Clinical methods: the history, physical, and laboratory examinations. 3rd edition. Boston: Butterworths; 1990.
35. Dorresteijn JA, Kriegsman DM, Assendelft WJ, et al. Patient education for preventing diabetic foot ulceration. Cochrane Database Syst Rev 2012;(10):CD001488.
36. Rogers LC, Frykberg RG, Armstrong DG, et al. The Charcot foot in diabetes. Diabetes Care 2011;34(9):2123–9.
37. Frykberg RG, Belczyk R. Epidemiology of the Charcot foot. Clin Podiatr Med Surg 2008;25(1):17–28, v.
38. Martinoli C, Court-Payen M, Michaud J, et al. Imaging of neuropathies about the ankle and foot. Semin Musculoskelet Radiol 2010;14(3):344–56.
39. Ahmad M, Tsang K, Mackenney PJ, et al. Tarsal tunnel syndrome: a literature review. Foot Ankle Surg 2012;18(3):149–52.
40. Delfaut EM, Demondion X, Bieganski A, et al. Imaging of foot and ankle nerve entrapment syndromes: from well-demonstrated to unfamiliar sites. Radiographics 2003;23(3):613–23.
41. Lee CH, Dellon AL. Prognostic ability of Tinel sign in determining outcome for decompression surgery in diabetic and nondiabetic neuropathy. Ann Plast Surg 2004;53(6):523–7 [cited 2013 Jun 15]. Available at: http://content. wkhealth.com/linkback/openurl?sid=WKPTLP:landingpage&an=00000637-200412000-00002.
42. Lifchez SD, Means KR, Dunn RE, et al. Intra- and inter-examiner variability in performing Tinel's test. J Hand Surg Am 2010;35(2):212–6 Elsevier Inc.
43. Abouelela A, Zohiery AK. The triple compression stress test for diagnosis of tarsal tunnel syndrome. Foot (Edinb) 2012;22(3):146–9 Elsevier Ltd.
44. Owens R, Gougoulias N, Guthrie H, et al. Morton's neuroma: clinical testing and imaging in 76 feet, compared to a control group. Foot Ankle Surg 2011;17(3): 197–200.
45. Dirim B, Resnick D, Ozenler NK. Bilateral Baxter's neuropathy secondary to plantar fasciitis. Med Sci Monit 2010;16(4):CS50–3.
46. Erra C, Granata G, Liotta G, et al. Ultrasound diagnosis of bony nerve entrapment: case series and literature review. Muscle Nerve 2013;48(3):1–20.
47. Krajewski KM, Lewis RA, Fuerst DR, et al. Neurological dysfunction and axonal degeneration in Charcot-Marie-Tooth disease type 1A. Brain 2000;123(Pt 7): 1516–27.

48. Lupski JR, Reid JG, Gonzaga-Jauregui C, et al. Whole-genome sequencing in a patient with Charcot-Marie-Tooth neuropathy. N Engl J Med 2010;362(13): 1181–91.
49. Yu JS, Cody ME. A template approach for detecting fractures in adults sustaining low-energy ankle trauma. Emerg Radiol 2009;16(4):309–18.
50. Dowling S, Spooner CH, Liang Y, et al. Accuracy of Ottawa ankle rules to exclude fractures of the ankle and midfoot in children: a meta-analysis. Acad Emerg Med 2009;16(4):277–87.
51. Bachmann LM, Kolb E, Koller MT, et al. Accuracy of Ottawa ankle rules to exclude fractures of the ankle and mid-foot: systematic review. BMJ 2003; 326(7386):417.
52. Leddy JJ, Kesari A, Smolinski RJ. Implementation of the Ottawa ankle rule in a university sports medicine center. Med Sci Sports Exerc 2002;34(1):57–62.
53. Wen DY. Risk factors for overuse injuries in runners. Curr Sports Med Rep 2007; 6(5):307–13.
54. Clemow C, Pope B, Woodall HE. Tools to speed your heel pain diagnosis. J Fam Pract 2008;57(11):714–23.
55. Yang J, Tibbetts AS, Covassin T, et al. Epidemiology of overuse and acute injuries among competitive collegiate athletes. J Athl Train 2012;47(2):198–204.
56. Coris EE, Lombardo JA. Tarsal navicular stress fractures. Am Fam Physician 2003;67(1):85–90.
57. Hall S, Lundeen G, Shahin A. Not just a sprain: 4 foot and ankle injuries you may be missing. J Fam Pract 2012;61(4):198–204.
58. el-Khoury GY, Dalinka MK, Alazraki N, et al. Chronic foot pain. ACR Appropriateness Criteria. Radiology 2000;215(Suppl):357–63.
59. Thomas JL, Christensen JC, Kravitz SR, et al. The diagnosis and treatment of heel pain: a clinical practice guideline—revision 2010. J Foot Ankle Surg 2010;49(Suppl 3):S1–19 Elsevier Ltd.
60. Kleipool RP, Blankevoort L. The relation between geometry and function of the ankle joint complex: a biomechanical review. Knee Surg Sports Traumatol Arthrosc 2010;18(5):618–27.
61. Kovaleski JE, Norrell PM, Heitman RJ, et al. Knee and ankle position, anterior drawer laxity, and stiffness of the ankle complex. J Athl Train 2008;43(3):242–8.
62. Johnston WL. Passive gross motion testing: Part I. Its role in physical examination. J Am Osteopath Assoc 1982;81(5):298–303.
63. Early J. Fractures and dislocations of the midfoot and forefoot. In: Bucholz R, Heckman J, Court-Brown C, editors. Rockwood & Green's fractures in adults. 6th edition. Philadelphia: Lippincott Williams; 2005. p. 2338–400.
64. Lim MR, Huang RC, Wu A, et al. Evaluation of the elderly patient with an abnormal gait. J Am Acad Orthop Surg 2007;15(2):107–17.
65. Oberg T, Karsznia A, Oberg K. Basic gait parameters: reference data for normal subjects, 10-79 years of age. J Rehabil R D 1993;30(2):210–23.
66. Petaros A, Slaus M, Coklo M, et al. Retrospective analysis of free-fall fractures with regard to height and cause of fall. Forensic Sci Int 2013;226(1–3):290–5 Elsevier Ireland Ltd.
67. Perron AD, Brady WJ. Evaluation and management of the high-risk orthopedic emergency. Emerg Med Clin North Am 2003;21(1):159–204.
68. Scolaro J, Ahn J, Mehta S. Lisfranc fracture dislocations. Clin Orthop Relat Res 2011;469(7):2078–80.

Gait
The Role of the Ankle and Foot in Walking

Andrew Dubin, MD, MS

KEYWORDS

- Gait • Ankle • Foot • Walking

KEY POINTS

- Common comorbidities that may hamper gait include, neurologic, orthopedic, cardiac, and pulmonary issues. As such, evaluation of gait and its associated deviations from normal requires an in-depth evaluation of the patient and an appreciation for the complexity of the task.
- Understanding gait starts with an appreciation of the basic determinants of gait. Functionally, the determinants of gait serve to optimize energy expenditure by either limiting the vertical excursion of the subject's center of gravity (COG), or optimizing stance phase limb position.
- Foot drop is a common gait deviation. It can result from a sciatic nerve neuropathy affecting the peroneal division, fibular nerve neuropathy at the level of the fibular head, or when symmetric, may be part of the manifestation of a polyneuropathy. Functionally, a foot drop results in a long limb. This will result in alterations of the gait cycle during swing phase.
- The common compensations for a foot drop include steppage gait, circumduction, and a persistently abducted limb. In all instances, these compensations serve to functionally shorten the long limb.
- Noninterventional options for management of common gait deviations secondary to ankle/foot dysfunction present challenges, but ultimately can be rewarding for both the patient and the treating physician. Before considering any treatment option, understanding the patient's needs and wishes is paramount.

For most people, walking, is a given and something that is taken for granted. It is a motor milestone that is typically acquired between 12 and 18 months of age. It is highly reproducible, with little variation in its subcomponents by 5 years of age.

Despite the outward appearance of simplicity, gait is a complex process. Many issues must be resolved for ambulation to become a practical form of mobility. Failure to meet certain criteria will typically result in people choosing alternate forms of mobility. The ankle–foot mechanism is a critical component of gait. The joints that comprise the ankle and the foot allow for full weight bearing through the stance phase

Department of PM&R, Albany Medical College, Albany, NY 12208, USA
E-mail address: dubina@mail.amc.edu

Med Clin N Am 98 (2014) 205–211
http://dx.doi.org/10.1016/j.mcna.2013.10.002
0025-7125/14/$ – see front matter © 2014 Elsevier Inc. All rights reserved.

limb, while at the same time dynamically adjusting to any alterations in terrain. The ability of the foot to adjust and respond to terrain perturbations optimizes people's ability to mobilize. Unfortunately, it also increases the risk of trauma to the ankle/foot mechanism.[1–4]

For ambulation to be considered the preferred form of mobility, several parameters need to be satisfied. They include: minimization of energy expenditure, maintenance of safety, and adequate speed to make walking practical over community-based distances; additionally, the activity must be painless. Failure to achieve any of these requirements will serve to either limit the distances walked, require the addition of an assistive device, or in extreme cases may cause to patient to choose an alternate form of mobility, such as a wheelchair or power-operated vehicle (POV). Common comorbidities that may hamper gait include, neurologic, orthopedic, cardiac, and pulmonary issues. As such, evaluation of gait and its associated deviations from normal requires an in-depth evaluation of the patient and an appreciation for the complexity of the task.[1,3,5]

Understanding gait starts with an appreciation of the basic determinants of gait. Functionally, the determinants of gait serve to optimize energy expenditure by either limiting the vertical excursion of the subject's center of gravity (COG), or optimizing stance phase limb position. A quick review of basic mechanics and physics reminds one that potential energy (PE) = mass × gravity × height (mgh). As such, anything that decreases the height function (vertical excursion) of the COG will conserve energy. The determinants of gait include, pelvic rotation, pelvic tilt, knee flexion at midstance, foot mechanisms, knee mechanisms, and lateral pelvic displacement. Pelvic rotation of $4°$ is responsible for functionally lengthening the swing phase limb, thereby preventing a sudden drop in the COG as the swing phase limb transitions to the stance phase limb. Pelvic tilt of 4 to $5°$ of the swing phase limb functionally lowers the COG, further decreasing its vertical excursion. The third determinant is knee flexion at stance (heel strike). Knee flexion in this case serves to decrease the vertical elevation of the COG during midstance, by shortening the hip to ankle distance. Additionally, this determinant will smooth the gait cycle by acting as a shock absorber at heel strike through eccentric loading of the quadriceps mechanism. It is critical to understand the role of eccentric loading during the gait cycle. From an energy expenditure standpoint, eccentric loading is an energy efficient form of muscle action. Foot mechanisms, from ankle dorsiflexion at heel strike to graded plantar flexion at foot flat, back to dorsiflexion at midstance and rollover, serve multiple purposes. The phase of heel strike to foot flat requires the ankle to progress from dorsiflexion to a plantar flexed posture. This serves to smooth the descent of the falling pelvis or COG. The controlled plantar flexion of the foot occurs through controlled eccentric action of the tibialis anterior as well as the common toe extensors and great toe extensor. The utilization of an eccentric action serves to minimize energy expenditure. Knee mechanisms serve to control the excursion of the COG. After midstance, the knee extends as the foot plantar flexes and supinates to lengthen the stance phase leg. This serves to lessen the fall of the pelvis at contralateral heel strike. The final determinant of gait is lateral displacement of the pelvis. This causes displacement of the COG toward the stance phase limb. This brings the COG over the base of support, in this case the stance phase foot. This serves to limit the activation of musculature needed to maintain stance phase stability. This last determinant serves to optimize the biomechanical function of the hip abductors, thereby minimizing energy expenditure. In summary, determinants 1 through 5 all reduce the vertical excursion of the COG. Determinant 6 controls the horizontal displacement of the COG, optimizing stance phase limb loading.[1,3,6–8]

GAIT DEVIATIONS IMPACTING ON ANKLE/FOOT MECHANISMS

Gait dysfunction can have an impact on one or many phases of the gait cycle. Deviations can have an impact on the stance phase or swing phase limb. Common gait deviations involving the ankle foot mechanism can profoundly influence the gait cycle, and result in fairly predictable compensations. Foot drop is a common gait deviation. It can result from a sciatic nerve neuropathy affecting the peroneal division, fibular nerve neuropathy at the level of the fibular head, or when symmetric, may be part of the manifestation of a polyneuropathy. Functionally, a foot drop results in a long limb. This will result in alterations of the gait cycle during the swing phase.[3,6,7,9]

A sciatic nerve neuropathy affecting the tibial division or a severe S 1 radiculopathy will result in weakness of the toe flexors, as well as the gastrocnemius and soleus muscles. Weakness of the soleus can significantly alter ankle/foot mechanisms. Functionally, the soleus serves to control the degree of tibial shank rollover during stance phase, as the stance phase limb progresses from foot flat to midstance. As the tibial shank progresses over a relatively plantar flexed ankle at foot flat to neutral position of the ankle at midstance, the soleus controls the rate of tibial shank progression via eccentric muscle action. Failure of soleus function results in excessive knee flexion with concomitant increase in energy expenditure owing to excessive fall of the COG during midstance. Additionally, excessive knee flexion results in further alteration in gait, as excessive concentric quadriceps activity is now required to control knee flexion. It is important to realize that concentric muscle actions, as opposed to eccentric muscle actions, are not energy conserving. As such, easy and early fatigue of the quadriceps muscle will be noted. This problem is frequently seen in patients who have a flexed knee deformity. Lastly, excessive knee flexion will increase compressive forces across the patellofemoral joint, fairly predictably resulting in anterior knee pain.[3,5–7,10,11]

A common issue involving the ankle foot mechanism may be one of pain secondary to degenerative joint disease of the true ankle joint, subtalar joint, or midfoot joints. In all instances, deviations of gait will occur. In this instance, the gait deviation will be limited to stance phase, and will universally result in a shortened stance time on the painful stance phase limb. As such, the swing phase time of the uninvolved limb will also be compromised, and the fluidity of the gait cycle will be compromised.[1,2,7,12]

A painful great toe metatarsal phalangeal joint will typically cause pain as the stance phase limb progresses from midstance to rollover. During slow walking, its impact on the gait cycle may be minimal. However, as ambulation velocities increase and the stance phase limb actively propels the COG forward, a blunting of rollover and premature initiation of swing phase will be noted. Subtalar joint issues do not typically impact on the stance phase of the gait cycle, unless ambulation is occurring on uneven terrain. In this instance, pain may now be appreciated, as the foot now has to move through ranges of hind foot valgus/varus and midfoot supination/pronation. As a result, alterations of stance phase time and compensations of how the foot articulates with the contact surface may occur.[1,2,7,12]

COMPENSATIONS FOR GAIT DEVIATIONS

The common compensations for a foot drop include steppage gait, circumduction, and a persistently abducted limb. In all instances, these compensations serve to functionally shorten the long limb. Steppage gait uses excessive hip and knee flexion on the involved side to shorten the limb. Circumduction and persistently abducted limb compensations shorten the long limb by moving the swing phase limb away from the midline of the body, with associated lateral trunk lean. All of these compensations alter gait mechanics and potentially increase energy expenditure. Steppage gait ambulation can be accomplished at community velocity, but will increase energy expenditure secondary to excessive hip and knee flexion. Circumduction and persistently abducted limb position, by the nature of the gait deviation, will predictably result in a slowed ambulation velocity and decreased energy expenditure. As such, these are commonly used deviations by the elderly or cardiopulmonary compromised patients with foot drop.

An interesting compensation for foot drop is vaulting. This compensation functionally lengthens the stance phase limb, as the patient gets up on his or her toes to clear the swing phase limb. This deviation serves to lengthen the stride length of the swing phase limb, but dramatically increases energy expenditure, as the COG will typically rise and fall 4 to 5 inches as opposed to the normal 2-inch excursion. This doubles energy expenditure for any given gait velocity. As such, this deviation is typically only used by young, fit, cardiopulmonary intact individuals who choose to maintain velocity at the expense of increased energy expenditure.[1-3,5-7]

Compensations for loss of soleal check revolve around stabilization of the knee during stance phase. This can include early and excessive activation of the quadriceps, or in some instances application of an external force on the anterior thigh to push the knee into extension. This is commonly done with the patient's ipsilateral hand pushing on the anterior thigh while weight bearing through the stance phase limb.[1,3,4]

Compensations for a painful true ankle joint, subtalar joint, midfoot joints, or great toe metatarsal phalangeal joint (MTP) joint arthritis all include shortening of the stance phase time. There are no other effective compensations the body can make. In this situation, modification of loading mechanics is the main compensatory strategy, which will typically be accomplished with an external bracing system.[1,3,4]

MANAGEMENT OF COMMON GAIT DEVIATIONS SECONDARY TO ANKLE FOOT DYSFUNCTION

Noninterventional options for management of common gait deviations secondary to ankle/foot dysfunction present challenges, but ultimately can be very rewarding for both the patient and the treating physician. Before considering any treatment option, understanding the patient's needs and wishes is paramount. Obtaining a history of vocational as well as avocational interests is mandatory. Appreciating the significance of underlying medical comorbidities is critical. Failure to appreciate the significance of the sensorily impaired foot can lead to catastrophic complications of skin breakdown and infection simply due to the wrong type or brace or foot orthotic being prescribed. Understanding the pathophysiology of the patient's foot deformity is also critical. Is this a static issue, or is the deformity going to progress as the disease process progresses?[11,13,14]

In all instances, orthotics can be thought of as either potentially load sharing, corrective, or accommodative. The style and materials used are determined in large part by the patient's needs, body habitus, and associated medical comorbidities.[2,7,11,13-16]

In the case of a foot drop, several factors need to be appreciated. First, one must address the etiology of the foot drop. Neurogenic etiologies may include peripheral causes such as inherited and acquired polyneuropathies, dense L 5 radiculopathy, common fibular nerve neuropathy at the fibular head, or a sciatic nerve common peroneal division neuropathy. Central nervous system disorders can also result in a foot drop posture secondary to gastrocnemius/soleus spasticity pulling the foot into an equinous posture. Common causes include cerebrovascular accident and multiple sclerosis. Primary muscle disorders such as distal myopathies including myotonic dystrophy and Myoshii myopathy can also cause a foot drop type posture. Duchennes and Beckers muscular dystrophy can also result in a foot drop type posture secondary to heel cord contracture. Mechanical dysfunction may also lead to a foot drop. This can be seen in patients with an anterior compartment syndrome, status postextensive debridement of the devitalized tibialis anterior muscle, resulting in mechanical loss of function. Each of these situations presents unique challenges and requires a thoughtful individualized approach.[6,7,11,14–16]

In both peripheral and central neurogenic causes, sensory examination is key. Loss of sensation along the dorsal and plantar surfaces must be noted if present. There is a high likelihood of significant sensory impairment in peripheral neurogenic causes. Additionally, in peripheral neurogenic causes, the foot drop is a flaccid foot drop, and as such, some way of maintaining the foot in dorsiflexion during swing phase and controlling the foot in stance phase is critical. In this scenario an ankle foot orthosis (AFO), although helpful for maintaining a plantar grade foot, requires certain modifications. A classic solid ankle polypropylene AFO may be contraindicated secondary to increased risk for skin breakdown, as it is an intimately fitting brace, with high pressure zones commonly noted at the level of the malleoli, navicular region, and base of the fifth metatarsal region. The rigid ankle, set at 90°, will also create potential issues during the gait cycle. With the ankle locked at 90°, excessive knee flexion is generated during stance phase. This can result in gait instability, increased risk of fall if there is quadriceps weakness, and increased energy expenditure by increasing the vertical excursion of the COG. A double metal upright AFO with a limited range of motion dorsiflexion spring assist ankle joint, affixed to a well configured soft leather upper shoe, via a split caliper, may be a much better option. In this case, the double metal upright removes pressure along the medial and lateral shin. The shoe made with a soft leather upper can be modified to an extradepth shoe to accommodate a custom insert to further disperse pressures over the sensory-impaired foot. The shoe should be constructed with a Blucher opening at the throat, as opposed to a Bal-Moral, to ease entrance into the shoe. The dorsiflexion spring assist optimizes foot position during swing phase and controls the loading response during stance phase, which in turn helps maintain knee stability.[11,13–16]

Central neurogenic causes of foot drop add the challenge of trying to control the foot while dealing with issues of plantar flexor spasticity. In these scenarios, plantar flexor spasticity is the generator of the foot drop posture and must be considered when prescribing an orthotic. Potential sensory impairment must be appreciated, but particular attention must be given to the issues of plantar flexor spasticity. If the spasticity is minimal and protective sensation is present, a standard plastic AFO with limited ankle range of motion will usually suffice. If the spasticity is severe and prevents placement of the involved foot in the AFO, and causes the foot to be maintained in a plantar flexed equinous posture, even in the AFO, then strong consideration needs to be given toward tone reduction. Botulinum toxin injections into the gastrocnemius/soleus complex may be very helpful and allow the foot to be brought to a plantar grade posture in the AFO. Heel cord lengthening procedures can be considered, with care taken to avoid overcorrection. This can result in loss of soleal check and lead to knee instability.

Primary muscle disorders resulting in a foot drop posture can be approached with an AFO. In these scenarios, early bracing to control the deforming forces is indicated, though the data are controversial. These patients will benefit from a limited range-of-motion AFO that limits plantar flexion to neutral and allows for free dorsiflexion. This type of brace at least theoretically will facilitate gastroc/soleus stretch and limit the development of a plantar flexion contracture. Mechanical dysfunction of dorsiflexion after anterior compartment syndrome with significant debridement of the tibialis anterior responds well to an AFO with a dorsiflexion spring assist. Molded plastic versus a double metal upright is determined by presence or absence of sensory impairment.

A sciatic neuropathy with involvement of the tibial division of the sciatic nerve presents interesting challenges. In isolation, the tibial nerve neuropathy proximal to the innervation of the posterior compartment of the lower leg results in loss of soleal check. This results in excessive knee flexion as the COG progresses over the stance phase limb from foot flat to midstance. This can be an underappreciated cause of increased risk to fall in the elderly. A chronic S 1 radiculopathy, not uncommonly seen in lumbar stenosis, can cause significant weakness of the gastroc/soleus complex. In this case, an AFO with limits placed on the degree of dorsiflexion permitted will be of utility. Typically, limiting dorsiflexion to 10° to 15° allows for functional rollover mechanics without resulting in knee instability. If the tibial neuropathy is part of a more diffuse sciatic neuropathy, a dorsiflexion spring assist, limited range-of-motion AFO will be very helpful.[11,13–16]

The painful arthritic ankle can also be treated with an AFO. In this case, the goal is to limit range of motion. As such, an intimately fitting plastic AFO may work well. Ankle range of motion should be limited to the painless part of the arc. If necessary, a solid ankle can be used, but consideration should be given to using it with a shoe that has a solid ankle cushion heel-type heel to smooth the gait cycle during stance phase and blunt excessive knee flexion. In instances of severe ankle pain with deformity that prevents full weight bearing, a patella tendon-bearing AFO can be fabricated. These types of bypass or load-sharing orthoses can de-weigh the lower leg from 10%, up to 100% when attached to a patten bottom. The painful arthritic subtalar joint can be treated with an AFO or a University California Biomechanics Laboratory (UCBL). The AFO is preferred when there are also issues that need to be addressed at the level of the true ankle joint. The UCBL is preferred in cases of isolated subtalar and hind foot pain, as it allows for excellent control of subtalar motion but does not restrict true ankle joint range.[10,13,15,16]

The painful great toe MTP joint can be managed with a custom insert that fits into the shoe and offloads the great toe during stance phase, particularly during rollover. In more severe cases, a rocker bottom shoe may be helpful, as it facilitates rollover mechanics without placing stress through the MTP joint of the great toe. Other options for managing the painful arthritic ankle, subtalar joint, or great toe MTP joint include single-crutch or cane-assisted ambulation. Both of these interventions can help partially de-weigh the stance phase limb, and to a minimal degree control rotatory forces at the subtalar joint. Typically, the crutch or the cane should be held in the contralateral hand, but in 50% of cases of a painful ankle or foot, the patient will use the assistive device long term on the ipsilateral side. The major restriction in using a crutch or a cane is that it limits upper extremity availability for carrying out activities of daily living that require bimanual use.[12,13,15,16]

REFERENCES

1. Murray MP, Drought AB, Kory RC. Walking patterns of normal men. J Bone Joint Surg Am 1964;46(2):335–60.
2. Murray MP. Gait as a total pattern of movement: including a bibliography on gait. Am J Phys Med 1967;46(1):290–333.
3. Winter DA. Biomechanics of normal and pathological gait: Implications for understanding human locomotor control. J Mot Behav 1989;21(4):337–55.

4. Buck P, Morrey BF, Chao EY. The optimum position of arthrodesis of the ankle. A gait study of the knee and ankle. J Bone Joint Surg Am 1987;69(7):1052–62.

5. Winters TF, Gage JR, Hicks R. Gait patterns in spastic hemiplegia in children and young adults. J Bone Joint Surg Am 1987;69:437–41.

6. Saunders JB, Inman VT, Eberhart HD. The major determinants in normal and pathological gait. J Bone Joint Surg Am 1953;35:543–58.

7. Fish DJ, Nielsen JP. Clinical assessment of human gait. JPO J Pract Orthod 1993; 5(2):39–48.

8. Pandy MG, Berme N. Quantitative assessment of gait determinants during single stance via three-dimensional model—part 1. Normal gait. J Biomech 1989; 22(6–7):717–24.

9. Rethlefsen S, Kay R, Dennis S, et al. The effects of fixed and articulated ankle-foot orthoses on gait patterns in subjects with cerebral palsy. J Pediatr Orthop 1999; 19(4):470–4.

10. Lehmann JF, Condon SM, Price R, et al. Gait abnormalities in hemiplegia: their correction by ankle-foot orthoses. Arch Phys Med Rehabil 1987;68(11):763–71.

11. Romkes J, Hell AK, Brunner R. Changes in muscle activity in children with hemi-plegic cerebral palsy while walking with and without ankle–foot orthoses. Gait Posture 2006;24(4):467–74.

12. Pandy MG, Berme N. Quantitative assessment of gait determinants during single stance viaa three-dimensional model—Part 2. Pathological gait. J Biomech 1989; 22(6–7):725–33.

13. Lehmann JF, Esselman PC, Ko MJ, et al. Plastic ankle-foot orthoses: evaluation of function. Arch Phys Med Rehabil 1983;64(9):402–7.

14. Geboers JF, Drost MR, Spaans F, et al. Immediate and long-term effects of ankle-foot orthosis on muscle activity during walking: a randomized study of patients with unilateral foot drop. Arch Phys Med Rehabil 2002;83(2):240–5.

15. Wong AM, Tang FT, Wu SH, et al. Clinical trial of a low-temperature plastic anterior ankle foot orthosis. Am J Phys Med Rehabil 1992;71(1):41–3.

16. Hsu JD, Michael JW, Fisk JR. American Academy of Orthopaedic Surgeons. AAOS atlas of orthoses and assistive devices. 4th edition. Philadelphia: Mosby; 2008. p. 326–8.

Nail and Skin Disorders of the Foot

Wesley W. Flint, MD, Jarrett D. Cain, DPM, MS*

KEYWORDS

- Onychomycosis • Onychocryptosis • Subungual tumors • Tinea pedis

KEY POINTS

- The dermal layers of the foot along with the nail possess properties that make the foot vulnerable to an array of disorders.
- These maladies are unique to the foot because of the extreme contact stresses it endures as well as the regular use of footwear, which maintains a moist environment.
- This damp climate allows for opportunistic infections and maceration of the skin.
- The foot is also prone to vascular disease given its distance from the heart and ascending venous drainage.

The dermal layers of the foot along with the nail possess properties that make it vulnerable to an array of disorders. These maladies are unique to the foot because of the extreme contact stresses it endures as well as the regular use of footwear, which maintains a moist environment. This damp climate allows for opportunistic infections and maceration of the skin. The foot is also prone to vascular disease given its distance from the heart and ascending venous drainage. This article reviews common conditions that afflict nail and dermal tissue of the foot.

NAIL DISORDERS

Nail disorders include disease that can be common and innocuous to subtle yet lethal. In this article we discuss some of the common disorders afflicting the nail and its supporting structures and a few conditions that should always be on the physician's differential.

The anatomy of the nail on the toe is similar to that of the finger. The nail is constructed of keratinized squamous cells.[1,2] The nail plate is a 3-layered keratin shield[3] that protects the distal pulp of the digit dorsally. It also acts to enhance the 2-point discrimination at the tip of the digit.[1] It is generated chiefly from the germinal matrix,

Neither author has any conflicts of interest to disclose.
Department of Orthopaedics, Penn State Hershey Medical Center, Penn State Bone and Joint Institute, 30 Hope Drive, Hershey, PA 17033, USA
* Corresponding author.
E-mail address: jcain1@hmc.psu.edu

which involves tissue lining the invaginated socket at the proximal aspect of the nail plate. The nail plate grows at a rate of 1 to 1.5 mm per month.[2] The germinal matrix gives rise to the more superficial layers of the nail. The nail is also created in part by the lunula and the sterile matrix, the former generating the middle portion and the latter interdigitating and supporting the deep surface.[2,3] The lunula is the white half circular structure deep to the nail plate and is the distal extent of the germinal matrix. When surgically ablating the nail, it is essential to excise the germinal matrix and lunula entirely to prevent remaining nail growth.

The eponychium is the area of the finger just proximal to the nail plate and includes the cuticle. The cuticle is the distal edge of the eponychium that lies over the nail at the proximal aspect and acts as a seal to the root of the nail.[2] The sterile matrix is a thin tissue just deep to the nail plate, which is adherent to not only the nail plate but also the deeper distal phalanx. Because of the intimate relationship between the sterile matrix and the distal phalanx, crush injuries that cause distal phalanx fractures also cause lacerations to occur at the sterile matrix. The nail plate can be dissected away from the nail plate in the case of a subungual hematoma and can be painful because of the pressure on the sterile matrix. The lateral edges of the nail plate are rolled into the tissue of the finger called the *paronychium*. This structure is prone to infection when it is disrupted due to trauma. It can also be involved in the case of onychocryptosis, commonly referred to as an *ingrown nail*. The distal nail plate is bordered by the hyponychium. The hyponychium creates a seal between the nail plate and the deeper, sensitive sterile matrix at the onychodermal band or solehorn.[2,3] The distal phalanx possesses a distal tuft that supports the sterile matrix and the adjacent nail plate.

Onychomycosis

Among the most chronic and common conditions at the nail is onychomycosis or fungal infestation of the nail. This affects approximately 6% to 13% of individuals (**Figs. 1 and 2**).[4] This fungal infestation leads to a thickened and brittle nail that is cosmetically disfiguring, particularly in middle-aged and elderly individuals. Functionally, it also can limit footwear and catch when pulling socks over the foot. The nail is discolored and can have white and yellow components. The dermis surrounding the nail is also hyperkeratotic. Rarely, this disorder can affect children and the hands. Risk factors include diabetes, family history, trauma, male sex, advanced age, tinea pedis, smoking, prolonged water exposure, and immunocompromised hosts.[5] The disorder is caused by a cast of fungal species, most commonly dermatophytes such as *Trichophyton rubrum* and *Trichophyton mentagrophytes*.[2,4,6] Less frequently, this infection can be caused by nondermatophytes and *Candida* species.[2]

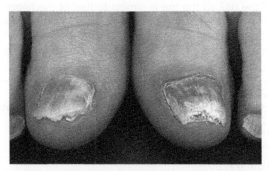

Fig. 1. Onychomycosis (*From* Hay R, Baran R. Onychomycosis: a proposed revision of the clinical classification. J Am Acad Dermatol 2011;65(6):1219–27.)

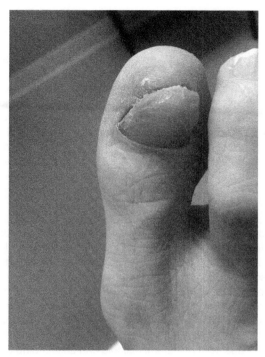

Fig. 2. Onychomycosis.

Great care must be taken when treating diabetic individuals because the dysmorphic nail may add contact stresses to the surrounding skin yielding a nonhealing ulceration. Professional nail care and close observation of these patients is necessary to avoid greater complications. Treatment can be limited to observation with periodic nail care.

Medical management of this disorder is frustrating. Antifungals must be taken for prolonged periods. Oral treatments may cause organ damage and may interact with other medications. Relapse risk is also high after medical management.[7] Topical regimens are also available; however, they are less effective, and the treatment time is greatly increased.[4] Current US Food and Drug Administration–approved regimens include Ciclopirox lacquer daily for 48 weeks; griseofulvin, 500 to 1000 mg daily until cleared; itraconazole, 200 mg daily for 12 weeks; and terbinafine, 250 mg daily for 12 weeks.[4] Terbinafine is the most effective treatment with cure rates around 76%.[7] Rarely, nail plate excision and matricectomies are performed if a nail poses a risk to surrounding soft tissues. Treatment may also be symptomatic, such as debridement of the nail and partial or total nail avulsion to avoid catching while donning footwear.[4]

Paronychia

Paronychia is a common infection involving the paronychium or lateral nail fold. This disorder is most common at the hallux in men in their third decade of life.[6] This occurs when the nail fold or cuticle is traumatized allowing for bacterial organisms enter and cause a pyogenic infection. Most frequent microbes include *Staphylococcus aureus;* however, *Streptococcus pyogenes, Pseudomonas, Proteus, Candida,* and oral flora may also be suspect.[8,9] Herpetic whitlow is a type of paronychia caused by herpes simplex virus.[9] Risk factors include picking soft tissues about the nails, hangnails, and trauma during pedicure. These can lead to a subungual abscess, chronic paronychia, cellulitis, and osteomyelitis or to a felon if not treated.[6,8]

Diagnosis is made by physical examination. The paronychium and/or cuticle are typically erythematous and painful with purulent drainage emanating from the junction of the nail plate and skin fold. Management includes Epson salt soaks if abscess is not suspected.[8] If an abscess is discovered on examination, simple local incision and drainage is performed leaving the wound open to drain. Antibiotic regimen should cover skin flora and pathogens that the individual may be exposed to such as *Pseudomonas* in case of prolonged water contact. Patients should be instructed to avoid future trauma to the cuticle and paronychial folds by trimming back hangnails with fingernail clippers.[8]

Onychocryptosis

Ingrown toenails or onychocryptosis is an exquisitely painful condition that is caused by a prominent lateral edge of the nail plate **Fig. 3**, which leads to dermal breakdown with inflammation at the lateral nail fold and, if not treated appropriately, to a pyogenic infection. This disorder occurs typically in males ages 15–40.[10] Onychocryptosis is instigated by either aberrant anatomy at the paronychium/nail junction, by improper nail care, or by crowding of the toes in cramped footwear. These allow for the nail edge to be driven deep within the periungual tissue causing inflammation.[11] Nonoperative management is warranted in early stages of onychocryptosis, including carefully lifting the sharp nail edge from the lateral nail fold and suspending the nail plate with a small piece of cotton. An individual may find this easiest after soaking the feet or bathing, when the nail fold is softened. With an acute painful episode, a metatarsal block with local anesthetic can be performed and the nail trimmed locally and elevated. If

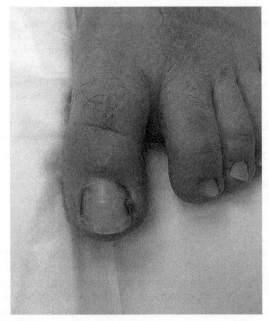

Fig. 3. Onychocryptosis.

simple excision of the nail spike is performed, it is necessary that the patient begin meticulous nail care to avoid recurrence of the ingrown nail.[10]

In the case of chronic onychocryptosis, a partial nail plate avulsion and partial ablation of the germinal matrix (matricectomy) is indicated **Fig. 4**. This is accomplished by performing a local block, splitting the nail plate longitudinally 2 to 3 mm from the affected corner of the nail with avulsion of this segment and either ablation or excision of the germinal matrix.[10,11] Ablation is completed with topical phenol or electrocautery. A recent Cochrane review found that ablation of the germinal matrix with phenol was more effective than partial surgical excision.[12] The authors also concluded that surgical management of chronic onychocryptosis was more effective than nonoperative treatment.[12] Complete removal of the nail plate and ablation of the germinal matrix may be warranted in cases of recurrent onychocryptosis. First-generation cephalosporins are typically prescribed postoperatively for 7 to 10 days.[6] Prevention is encouraged by proper nail care by cutting the nail perpendicular to the axis of the toe, leaving the lateral and medial edges of the nail plate to extend beyond the distal extent of the lateral nail fold.

Subungual Hematoma and Sterile Matrix Lacerations

Trauma to the sterile matrix of the nail is a common occurrence. These are simple to manage in the office or in an emergency department setting. Usually subungual hematomas and lacerations to the sterile matrix occur when the distal aspect of the phalanx sustains a violent compressive force, such as dropping a canned food item on an unshod foot. Although uncommon, one must always consider subungual melanoma in the differential of a darkly pigmented lesion deep to a nail.[6] A general rule is that if the subungual hematoma involves greater than 50% of the subungual space without fracture of the tuft of the distal phalanx, removal of the nail plate and primary repair of

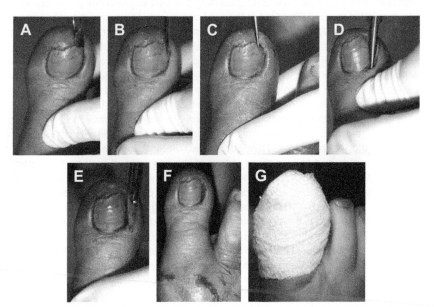

Fig. 4. (*A–G*) Treatment of onychocryptosis. (*From* Coughlin MJ, Saltzman CL, Anderson RB. Mann's surgery of the foot and ankle. Philadelphia: Saunders, an imprint of Elsevier Inc; 2014.)

the sterile matrix is indicated, as there is a high likelihood of laceration.[1] A recent review refuted this claim and found that most patients without fracture and subungual hematoma greater than 50% recovered with few nail deformities with simple trephination.[13] Failure to repair the matrix laceration can lead to a deformed nail that may not adhere normally to the matrix.[1]

Trephination is warranted in subungual hematomas that are painful. They reduce pain by decompressing the subungual space and limit pressure necrosis of the sterile matrix in an acute setting. It is essential that radiographs are taken of the affected digit to rule out a tuft fracture of the distal phalanx before proceeding. Trephination is performed by making a small burr hole with a stout hypodermic needle (18 or 20 gauge), scalpel, a small biopsy punch, or a disposable battery-powered cautery device.[14] Numerous devices and methods have been described to perform this procedure. The hole created should only penetrate the nail plate to allow for evacuation of the hematoma. Trephination with a small 2-mm biopsy punch is optimal, as it is atraumatic to the underlying matrix and avoids cauterization of the blood within the hematoma to allow for more effective drainage.[14] If a distal phalanx fracture on radiograph is present with a subungual hematoma, this constitutes an open fracture, which necessitates urgent debridement, irrigation, and repair. The administration of antibiotics is debatable. Some surgeons elect to treat with intravenous antibiotics in the acute setting and others would argue that thorough debridement and irrigation only are necessary.[1,6] Cefazolin in most cases is the preferred choice with clindamycin being a suitable alternative in case of sensitivity to cephalosporins. Antibiotics are typically administered immediately after the discovery of an open fracture.

Our preferred technique is to administer intravenous antibiotics and update tetanus prophylaxis as soon as possible. We then perform a metatarsal block with 1% lidocaine and 0.25% bupivacaine, which are injected dorsally at the level of the distal metatarsal directed plantarly to block the common digital nerves and their proper digital branches to the affected toe after cleansing the skin with alcohol pads. Generally, 10 mL of solution is used. The foot is then prepared with either chlorhexidine or povidone iodine solution. We prefer to use a surgical scrub brush as this is applied. A sterile field with towels is then created. We find it helpful to then create a small tourniquet with a rolled up finger from a sterile surgical glove or a Penrose drain tied over the proximal aspect of the digit. The nail is carefully elevated with a pair of tenotomy scissors directed distal to proximal, under and parallel to the nail plate. The nail plate is then elevated by placing the blades of the scissors in a closed fashion between the layers and spreading the scissors apart in a gentle fashion to release the sterile matrix from the undersurface of the nail plate. Caution must be used, as this can cause iatrogenic laceration to the matrix. This is continued under the entirety of the nail plate to the germinal matrix and to the lateral extent of the nail plate. It may be necessary to release the tissue dorsally between the nail plate and the eponychium or cuticle proximally to the germinal matrix. This dorsal release is also performed in the same fashion by spreading apart the tenotomy scissors after placing them in a closed fashion between the tissue layers. The nail should then be free and the nail plate can be grasped with a small hemostat and removed. The underlying sterile matrix is then irrigated with at least 1000 mL of sterile saline in an unpressurized fashion. The sterile matrix is then inspected and debrided of small free pieces of bone and hematoma. The lacerated edges of the sterile matrix are then re-approximated with 5–0 chromic gut suture anatomically in an interrupted fashion. Any other lacerations about the toe are then closed with 4–0 nylon suture in an interrupted fashion. It is then necessary to place something between the dorsal and deep layers of the germinal matrix. A variety of materials can be used to place in the germinal matrix including intravenous drip chamber or foil from petrolatum gauze packaging to name a few. We prefer to use the native nail plate as a spacer to prevent adhesion at the germinal matrix. The nail plate is debrided of any soft tissue and cleansed if necessary. Provisionally, the nail is replaced and marked for suture placement. We then use a 4–0 or 3–0 nylon suture to secure the nail plate. The suture is placed 3 to 4 mm proximal to the eponychium and into the space between the opposing germinal matrix layers where the nail plate resides. The suture is then placed superficial to deep at one corner of the proximal aspect of the nail and then deep to superficial through the other corner of the nail. The suture is then placed deep to superficial through the eponychium and the opposite corner of the toe to create a mattress suture through the nail plate. This suture is later cut and the nail plate is allowed to fall off after the new nail begins to grow and the sterile matrix laceration has healed. We discharge patients with a 5- to 7-day supply of first-generation cephalosporins orally or clindamycin. Wound care includes keeping the foot clean and dry and performing daily or twice-daily dry dressing changes.

SUBUNGUAL TUMORS
Glomus Tumor

A tumor that is sensitive to temperature fluctuation is pathognomonic for a glomus tumor. Glomus tumors are rare, representing 1.5% of benign soft tissue tumors of the extremities, and typically affect the hands in 75% of cases.[15] They occur between ages 30 to 50.[15] They originate from the glomus body, a thermoregulatory apparatus at the distal digit.[15] These lesions present as a triad of pain, point tenderness, and temperature sensitivity.[15] These masses are typically worked up with magnetic resonance imaging showing the location of the mass. The magnetic resonance image appearance is dark on T1 and bright on T2.[15] Masses have a characteristic purplish hue to grey-pink and are 1 to 2 mm in diameter.[6,15] Excision of the mass is warranted for pain relief. Recurrence rate is between 4% and 15%.[15]

Subungual Exostosis

Subungual exostoses are benign lesions that lift the nail from the sterile matrix and impede the patient from donning footwear. These masses are uncommon and typically occur in the third and fourth decades of life.[16] The great toe is involved 75% of the time[17]; however, subungual exostoses can occur on any digit.[16] The etiology is thought to be an inciting trauma or infection that initiates reparative mechanisms within the distal phalanx where metaplasia leads to an abnormal bony growth.[16,17] Clinically, the lesion appears as fullness beneath the nail. Radiographically, they originate from the dorsal surface of the distal phalanx.[16] Treatment includes excision with repair of the nail and sterile matrix. The recurrence rate is between 6% and 12%.[17]

Subungual Osteochondroma

A mimicking lesion to subungual exostosis is an osteochondroma. Osteochondroma at the distal phalanx occurs in men, usually around the second decade of life.[16] The presentation is similar to subungual exostosis, although the mass originates near the physis at the proximal aspect of the distal phalanx.[16] Another major difference between the 2 lesions is that the osteochondroma possesses a hyaline cartilaginous cap in which the subungual exostosis possesses a fibrocartilagenous cap.[16] Treatment is the same.

Subungual Melanoma

Subungual melanoma is a severe variant of malignant melanoma with a subtle presentation. This disorder represents 1% of melanoma cases and carries a 16% to

80% survival rate at 5 years.[6,18] Subungual melanoma is most often found in African and Asian patients.[6,18] Up to 20% of subungual lesions are amelanotic, making the diagnosis challenging.[6] Median age at presentation is in the sixth to seventh decades of life and does not have a sex preference.[2,6] Diagnostic clues include Hutchinson's sign, or the extension of melanotic pigment into the nail folds.[2] Longitudinal melanonychia, which is a dark longitudinal stripe at the nail, may also be a clue to diagnosis; however, this may be present in other benign processes.[2] Treatment is controversial. It is unclear whether local excision, including Mohs micrographic excision, versus wide excision is most advantageous, although there is a trend toward partial digit-sparing surgery.[6,18] The key to survival is prompt diagnosis and treatment.

Acral Melanoma

Acral Melanoma is another mimicking lesion that is potentially fatal that resembles a simple subungual hematoma, ulcerations, or other benign skin lesions. Practitioners must have a high level of suspicion to discover these lesions, as they do not occur typically in lightly pigmented individuals with a history of high level of sun exposure.

SKIN DISORDERS
Cellulitis

Cellulitis is most often the result of breaches in skin integrity and is associated with risk factors such as obesity, venous insufficiency, diabetic foot ulcers, or lymphatic disruption from prior surgery **Fig. 5**.[19] Clinical presentation includes areas of edema, warmth, tenderness, and redness. Along with the clinical presentation, laboratory values of complete blood count, erythrocyte sedimentation rate, and C-reactive protein should be obtained. Blood cultures and wound cultures, if an open wound is present, may be necessary.

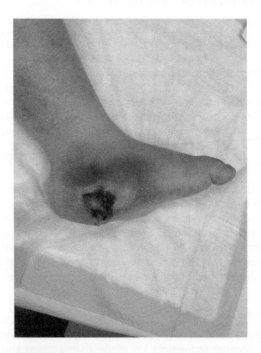

Fig. 5. Cellulitis.

Oral and intravenous antibiotic therapy is administered according to the causative organism, which is most commonly gram-positive bacteria. First-line therapy is medical, and initial antimicrobial agents should include coverage of *Streptococci* and *Staphylococci* in the setting of trauma.[20]

Tinea Pedis

Tinea pedis is a superficial fungal infection that affects the plantar sole and the interdigital spaces of the foot. Commonly known as *athletes' foot*, the disorder affects individuals with increased contact with swimming pools, athletic shoes, and sports equipment and, to a lesser degree, those with depressed immune function.[21,22] Clinically, this condition presents in the form of interdigital, moccasin, and vesiculobullous changes. Interdigital tinea pedis is the most common form with the appearance of macerated skin with fissures and often erythema (**Fig. 6**). Moccasin tinea pedis presents as scaling plaques with a mildly erythematous base on the heels, soles, and lateral aspects of the feet, whereas vesiculobullous lesions have the appearance of vesicles with multiple blisters with erythema.[23] Although interdigital tinea pedis is caused by T rubrum, more aggressive forms of tinea are caused by T *mentagrophytes* with pain, erosions, foul odor, macerations, and fissures commonly in conjunction with a superimposed bacterial infection.[9] Diagnosis is often based on clinical examination in combination with microscopic examination of potassium hydroxide skin samples of the lesion border that will appear as multiple, branched, septate hyphae.[24]

Treatment of tinea pedis involves topical medications with the goals of eradication or inhibition of the growth of the fungal infection. Topical antifungal medications such as azoles, allylamines, and thiocarbamates are effective in the treatment of interdigital tinea pedis. Oral terbinafine has been reported to have greater efficacy than azole medications.[25] If erythema secondary from bacterial infection is present, treatment may also involve an oral antibiotic. Moccasin and vesiculobullous tinea pedis can be more resistant to topical therapy that is more effective against interdigital tinea pedis, however, may require more aggressive systemic antifungal treatment. These treatments carry the risk of hepatotoxicity.[26] Oral or systemic management must be combined with other conservative treatment in the form of antimoisture socks, antifungal powders, and proper shoegear in public bathrooms, gyms, and showers.

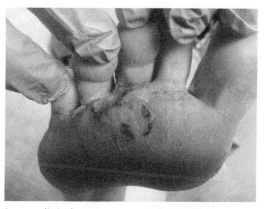

Fig. 6. Interdigital tinea pedis is the most common form with the appearance of macerated skin with fissures and often erythema.

This management is advised to prevent recurrence secondary to fungal spores that are prevalent in moist environments.

Verrucae Vulgaris

Verrucae are a particular type of virus that cause warts on the plantar aspect of the foot. The virus is usually caused by the human papillomavirus, particularly types 1, 2, and 3 **Fig. 7**.[27] Clinical presentation includes hyperkeratosis, callous lesions on the plantar aspect of the foot with focal tenderness on direct palpation or upon weight-bearing in shoes. Because of the hyperkeratotic appearance of the lesions, they are often dismissed as callous secondary to biomechanics of the foot; however, upon debridement, the lesions reveal pinpoint hemorrhaging or punctate black dots that are thrombosed capillary vessels.[28]

Treatment for verrucae consists of destructive therapies including cryotherapy with liquid nitrogen, local curettage, and electrodessication. Topical treatments such as salicyclic acid preparations, podophyllotoxin, retinoids, silver nitrate, and immuno-therapeutic agents (squaric acid dibutylester) have also been described.[27] Oral cimet-idine has been found to be effective alone or in combination with topical medication.[29] Although topical, oral, and destructive treatments are effective, recurrence of this condition is common.

Porokeratosis

Porokeratosis is a skin disorder that commonly presents on the plantar aspect of the foot with hyperkeratosis and a clear isolated lesion with central depression and raised rolled borders that are painful on weightbearing **Fig. 8**.[30] This condition was first described by Taub and Steinberg in 1970.[31] They described the lesion as

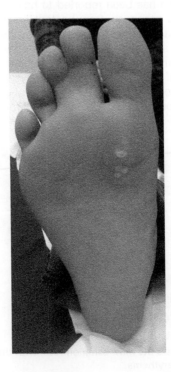

Fig. 7. Verrucae Vulgaris.

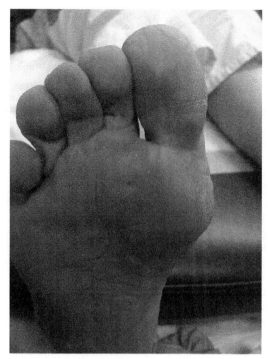

Fig. 8. Porokeratosis.

a hyperkeratotic lesion that was closely related to eccrine glands of the foot, typically found over pressure points on the plantar aspect.[31] Their relation to the eccrine gland has been disputed.[32,33] It was most commonly found in adults and in women 75% of the time.[31] The lesion possesses a hyperkeratotic plug that penetrates deep into the foot.[31–34] Unlike verrucae, it does not contain capillaries that give the characteristic pinpoint bleeding during debridement.[34] Treatments with high success rates include excision of the painful lesion with a #15 scalpel blade, sclerosing agents such as 2% to 4% alcohol solution with local anesthetic, and cryotherapy.[31,33,34]

SUMMARY

Disorders of the dermis and the nails on the feet are common. Despite the simplicity of the skin and nail disorders of the foot, they can be debilitating and impact the patient's ability to ambulate and perform activities of daily living. Diagnosis in most cases is confirmed on physical examination alone. Diligent care of skin and nail disorders can prevent further pathology involving the deeper structures of the foot and allow the patient to fully participate in their usual activities.

REFERENCES

1. Wang QC, Johnson BA. Fingertip injuries. Am Fam Physician 2011;63:1961–6.
2. Mayeaux EJ. Nail disorders. Prim Care 2000;27:333–51.
3. DeOrio JK, Coughlin MJ. Toenail abnormalities. In: Coughlin MJ, Mann RA, Saltzman CL, editors. Surgery of the foot and ankle. 8th edition. Philadelphia: Mosby Elsevier; 2007. p. 738–9.

4. Gupta AK, Tu LQ. Therapies for onychomycosis: a review. Dermatol Clin 2006;24: 375–9.
5. Gupta AK, Cooper EA. Onychomycosis. In: Williams H, Bigby M, editors. Evidence-based dermatology. 2nd edition. Maulden (MA): Blackwell; 2008. p. 362–86.
6. Weinfeld SB. Nail and skin disorders of the foot and ankle. In: Michael SP, editor. OKU foot and ankle. 4th edition. Rosemont (IL): American Academy of Orthopaedic Surgeons; 2008.
7. Gupta AK, Ryder JE, Johnson AM. Cumulative metaanalysis of systemic antifungal agents for the treatment of onychomycosis. Br J Dermatol 2000;150: 537–44.
8. Rigopoulos D, Larios G, Gregoriou S. Acute and chronic paronychia. Am Fam Physician 2008;77:339–46.
9. Hsu AR, Hsu JW. Topical review: infections in the foot and ankle patient. Foot Ankle Int 2012;33:612–9.
10. Park DH, Singh D. Clinical review: the management of ingrowing toenails. BMJ 2012;344:e2089.
11. Heidlebaugh JJ, Lee H. Management of the ingrown toenail. Am Fam Physician 2009;79:303–8, 311–12.
12. Eekhof JA, Van Wijk B, Knuitstingh NA, et al. Interventions for ingrowing toenails. Cochrane Database Syst Rev 2012;(4):CD001541.
13. Batrick N, Hashemi K, Freij R, et al. Treatment of uncomplicated subungual hematoma. Emerg Med J 2003;20:65.
14. Khan MA, West E, Tyler M. Two millimeter biopsy punch: a painless and practical instrument for evacuation of subungual haematomas in adults and children. J Hand Surg Eur Vol 2011;36:615–7.
15. Pater TJ, Marks RM. Glomus tumor of the hallux: case presentation and review of the literature. Foot Ankle Int 2004;25:434–7.
16. Lee SK, Moon SJ, Lee YH, et al. Two distinctive subungual pathologies: subungual exostosis and subungual osteochondroma. Foot Ankle Int 2007;28:595–601.
17. Williard KJ, Cappel MA, Kozin SH, et al. Benign subungual tumors. J Hand Surg 2012;37:1276–86.
18. Martin DE, English JC, Goitz RJ. Subungual malignant melanoma. J Hand Surg 2011;36:704–7.
19. Stevens DL, Bisno AL, Chambers HF, et al. Practice guidelines for the diagnosis and management of skin and soft-tissue infections. Clin Infect Dis 2005;41: 1373–406.
20. Anakwenze OA, Milby AH, Gans I, et al. Foot and ankle infections: diagnosis and management. J Am Acad Orthop Surg 2012;20:684–93.
21. Brenner IK, Shek PN, Shepard RJ. Infections in athletes. Sports Med 1994;17: 86–107.
22. Wolff K, Johnson RA, Suurmond D. Cutaneous fungal infections. In: Seils A, Englis MR, editors. Fitzpatrick's color atlas, synopsis of clinical dermatology. 5th edition. New York: McGraw-Hill; 2005. p. 686–98.
23. Field LA, Adams BB. Tinea pedis in athletes. Int J Dermatol 2008;47:485–92.
24. Pecci M, Comeau D, Chawla V. Skin conditions in the athlete. Am J Sports Med 2009;37:406–18.
25. Bell-Syer SE, Hart R, Crawford F, et al. Oral treatments for fungal infections of the skin of the foot. Cochrane Database Syst Rev 2002;(2):CD003584.
26. Shear NH. Review: oral antifungal therapy has low risk for adverse events in superficial dermatophytosis and onychomycosis. ACP J Club 2008;148:14.

27. Micali G, Dall'Oglio F, Nasca MR, et al. Management of cutaneous warts: an evidence-based approach. Am J Clin Dermatol 2004;5:311–7.
28. Pharis DB, Teller C, Wolf JE. Cutaneous manifestations of sports participation. J Am Acad Dermatol 1997;36:448–59.
29. Simonart T, de Maertelaer V. Systemic treatments for cutaneous warts: a systematic review. J Dermatolog Treat 2012;23:72–7.
30. Himmelstein R, Lynnfield MR. Punctate porokeratosis. Arch Dermatol 1984;120: 263–4.
31. Taub J, Steinberg MD. Porokeratosis plantaris discrete, a previously unrecognized dermatopathological entity. Int J Dermatol 1970;9:83–90.
32. Dockery GL. Evaluation and treatment of metatarsalgia and keratotic disorders. In: Myerson MS, editor. Foot and ankle disorders, vol. 1. Philadelphia: WB Saunders; 2000. p. 364.
33. Mandojana RM, Katz R, Rodman OG. Porokeratosis planatris discreta. J Am Acad Dermatol 1984;10:679–82.
34. Limmer BL. Cryosurgery of porokeratosis plantaris discreta. Arch Dermatol 1979; 115:582–3.

Hallux Valgus

Paul J. Hecht, MD*, Timothy J. Lin, MD

KEYWORDS

- Bunion • Hallux valgus • Metatarsus primus varus

KEY POINTS

- Hallux valgus is a common progressive forefoot deformity that affects women more commonly than men.
- Tight-fitting and high-heeled shoes, gender, and genetics seem to be the most important predisposing factors.
- Treatment consists of footwear modification and surgical procedures, depending on the patient's symptoms and the severity of the deformity.
- Radiographic evaluation must include weight-bearing radiographs.

INTRODUCTION

Hallux valgus is the most common problem of the forefoot in adults.[1] The deformity of hallux valgus is progressive, and involves several stages, but begins with lateral deviation of the great toe (hallux) and medial deviation of the first metatarsal (metatarsus primus varus).[2] In its later stages, hallux valgus involves progressive subluxation of the first metatarsophalangeal (MTP) joint.[1] The cause of hallux valgus has been debated for years, but is likely associated with genetic predisposition, restrictive footwear, other foot deformities such as pronation of the hindfoot[3] and pes planus (flatfoot),[1] hypermobility, contracture of the Achilles tendon, and neuromuscular disorders such as cerebral palsy and stroke.[4,5] No association has been made between hallux valgus and either obesity or occupation (except for ballet dancing).[1,6,7]

Adults are more commonly affected than children, although juvenile hallux valgus does occur. Women are diagnosed more frequently than men, with a ratio as high as 15:1 in some studies,[8] and require surgery more often, which is thought to be associated with differential use of tight-fitting and high-heeled shoes. Women also tend to have higher rates of ligamentous laxity and different bony anatomy that may play a role.[9]

Disclosures: None.
Department of Orthopaedic Surgery, Dartmouth Hitchcock Medical Center, One Medical Center Drive, Lebanon, NH 03756, USA
* Corresponding author.
E-mail address: paul.j.hecht@hitchcock.org

Med Clin N Am 98 (2014) 227–232
http://dx.doi.org/10.1016/j.mcna.2013.10.007
0025-7125/14/$ – see front matter Published by Elsevier Inc.
medical.theclinics.com

Symptoms of hallux valgus include poor-fitting shoes, plantar foot pain, medial first MTP joint pain, deep MTP aching pain from joint degeneration, and pain with weight bearing.

Management of hallux valgus generally begins with conservative (nonoperative) treatment, especially in juvenile hallux valgus, the elderly, or patients with significant comorbidities. Conservative modalities include avoidance of tight-fitting, high-heeled shoes; wearing wide-toed soft footwear; use of various inserts/pads; and physical therapy. Surgical correction is indicated in situations of failed nonoperative management, progressive, painful deformity, and disruption of lifestyle and/or activity.

DIAGNOSIS

Evaluation of the patient with suspected hallux valgus should include a thorough history, including any pertinent family history; physical examination; and radiologic examination with weight-bearing radiographs. History should focus on duration of symptoms, activity modification, footwear, and types of any previous interventions. Physical examination must include observation of gait, alignment, and range of motion of the first MTP joint and of both lower extremities, and examination of the bare feet both with weight bearing and without. Special attention should be paid to type and wear pattern of footwear; specific areas of pain and tenderness; the presence of calluses or corns; deformities of the lesser toes, midfoot, or hindfoot; laxity of the first ray (from the great toe to the hindfoot); the presence of a large bunion; and the presence or absence of Achilles tightness.

PATHOGENESIS/PROGRESSION

The first ray bears a significant amount of weight as it maintains the position of the medial arch.[10] Any deformity that disrupts the integrity of the first ray can lead to hallux valgus.[5] As seen in **Table 1**,[5] there is a series of steps in the progression of hallux valgus, but the steps are not necessarily followed in a specific order. Because the medial structures of the first MTP joint are weak, including the medial collateral ligament and the medial sesamoid bone, they tend to fail first.[11] The metatarsal head eventually drifts medially, the proximal phalanx shifts into valgus, the bursa of the medial eminence becomes inflamed and prominent, and the extensor hallucis longus and flexor hallucis longus tendons bowstring laterally, exaggerating the deformity.[5,12,13]

Table 1 The multiple steps that are involved in the progression of hallux valgus (not necessarily in order)	
Potential Causes of Hallux Valgus	
Extrinsic Factors	**Intrinsic Factors**
Footwear (high heels, narrow shoes)	Genetics
Excess weight bearing	Sex (female>male)
	Ligamentous laxity
	Other foot deformities (pes planus, hindfoot pronation, metatarsus primus varus)
	Age
	Neuromuscular disorders (eg, cerebral palsy, stroke)

Data from Perera AM, Mason L, Stephens MM. The pathogenesis of hallux valgus. J Bone Joint Surg Am 2011;93(17):1650–61.

CLASSIFICATION

Severity of hallux valgus is typically based on symptoms and radiologic assessment using weight-bearing radiographs and is described as mild, moderate, or severe. Two angles of importance in the assessment of radiologic severity of hallux valgus are the hallux valgus angle (HVA; normal <15°)[2] and intermetatarsal angle (IMA; normal <9°).[4] Classification of hallux valgus is based on the HVA and IMA, and this is summarized in **Fig. 1** and **Table 2**.

TREATMENT
Nonoperative Treatment

Conservative interventions should be used before surgical intervention, and should be the mainstay of treatment in juvenile hallux valgus,[14] the elderly, and patients with severe neuropathy or other comorbidities that make them poor surgical candidates. The goal of conservative management should be to decrease severity of symptoms and avoid lifestyle/activity modifications because there is no evidence to show that nonoperative therapies have the ability to correct the hallux valgus deformity.

Patients should first be counseled to avoid using tight-fitting or high-heeled footwear. They should be advised to seek out soft, wide-toed footwear in order to attempt to slow progression. Various inserts have been used in order to alleviate pain, including hallux valgus splints, bunion shields (**Fig. 2**), toe spacers, and night splints.

However, orthotics have not been shown to prevent or slow progression of hallux valgus.[15] In one recent study published in 2013 by Reina and colleagues[16] there

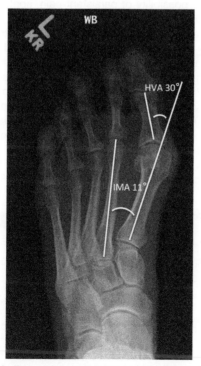

Fig. 1. Mild to moderate hallux valgus. HVA is 30° and the IMA is 11°. The first MTP joint is congruent, but there is a large exostosis over the medial aspect of the first metatarsal head that is associated with an overlying soft tissue prominence.

Table 2
The classification of hallux valgus based on standing anteroposterior (AP) radiographs

	Radiographic Classification of Hallux Valgus		
	HVA (°)	IMA (°)	Subluxation of Lateral Sesamoid on AP View (%)
Normal	<15	<9	—
Mild	<20	≤11	<50
Moderate	20–40	<16	50–75
Severe	>40	≥16	>75

was no difference in progression of radiographic severity of hallux valgus (measured by HVA and IMA) in 54 women randomized to custom-made orthotics versus no treatment at 12-month follow-up. Given the unpredictability of outcome with regard to activity tolerance and pain after surgical correction, patients who are able to maintain a high level of sport or activity should prolong surgery until this is not the case.

Over-the-counter antiinflammatory medications, acetaminophen, and (rarely) injections may be used to alleviate pain.

Operative Treatment

Preoperative counseling is important when considering operative correction. Patients should be warned of the possibility of persistent pain, continued need for footwear modification, and risk of recurrence, as well as general risks of surgery and anesthesia.

More than 140 surgical procedures have been described to correct hallux valgus, but no single procedure has been shown to lead to improved outcomes. Procedures are generally grouped into categories, each of which is used as indicated based on severity of disease with respect to radiographic parameters, presence or absence of significant first MTP joint degeneration, and whether or not the deformity is passively correctable by the examiner. General categories include distal soft tissue procedures, first metatarsal osteotomies, proximal phalanx osteotomies, arthrodesis (fusion), and resection arthroplasties. Some combination of these procedures is commonly used to treat patients.

Juvenile hallux valgus is best treated conservatively for as long as possible, given the increased risk of recurrence, shown to be as high as 40% to 60% in one series

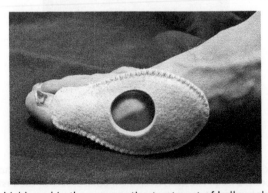

Fig. 2. A bunion shield used in the conservative treatment of hallux valgus.

of 21 bunions in 13 adolescents treated operatively.[17] There is also a higher risk of overcorrection with surgical management in skeletally immature patients.[18]

SUMMARY

Hallux valgus is a common foot problem whose cause and progression is multifactorial, complex, and poorly known. It is likely related primarily to genetic predisposition and use of tight, constrained footwear. Hallux valgus shows a predilection toward women, although this may also be related to differences in shoe preferences between sexes. It is a progressive disorder with no treatment known to slow or stop progression. Shoe inserts can be used as a conservative measure with unpredictable efficacy. Surgery is indicated in healthy individuals when nonoperative measures fail, although outcomes from surgery are not always predictable. Adverse effects of surgery include infection and recurrence. Many procedures have been described in the literature, including soft tissue and bony reconstruction of the first ray. The procedure that is indicated depends on the severity of the deformity.

REFERENCES

1. Mann RA, Coughlin MJ. Hallux valgus–etiology, anatomy, treatment and surgical considerations. Clin Orthop Relat Res 1981;(157):31–41.
2. Hardy RH, Clapham JC. Observations on hallux valgus; based on a controlled series. J Bone Joint Surg Br 1951;33(3):376–91.
3. Inman VT. Hallux valgus: a review of etiologic factors. Orthop Clin North Am 1974; 5(1):59–66.
4. Mann R, Coughlin M. Adult hallux valgus, surgery of the foot and ankle, 1. St Louis (MO): CV Mosby; 1993. p. 204–16.
5. Perera AM, Mason L, Stephens MM. The pathogenesis of hallux valgus. J Bone Joint Surg Am 2011;93(17):1650–61.
6. Einarsdottir H, Troell S, Wykman A. Hallux valgus in ballet dancers: a myth? Foot Ankle Int 1995;16(2):92–4.
7. Hung LK, Ho YF, Leung PC. Survey of foot deformities among 166 geriatric inpatients. Foot Ankle 1985;5(4):156–64.
8. Pique-Vidal C, Sole MT, Antich J. Hallux valgus inheritance: pedigree research in 350 patients with bunion deformity. J Foot Ankle Surg 2007;46(3):149–54.
9. Wilkerson RD, Mason MA. Differences in men's and women's mean ankle ligamentous laxity. Iowa Orthop J 2000;20:46–8.
10. McBride ED. A conservative operation for bunions. J Bone Joint Surg 1928; 10(735):14.
11. Wilson DW. Treatment of hallux valgus and bunions. Br J Hosp Med 1980;24(6): 548–9.
12. Haines RW, Mc DA. The anatomy of hallux valgus. J Bone Joint Surg Am 1954; 36(2):272–93.
13. Piggott H. The natural history of hallux valgus in adolescence and early adult life. J Bone Joint Surg Br 1960;42(4):749–60.
14. Omey ML, Micheli LJ. Foot and ankle problems in the young athlete. Med Sci Sports Exerc 1999;31(Suppl 7):S470–86.
15. Torkki M, Malmivaara A, Seitsalo S, et al. Surgery vs orthosis vs watchful waiting for hallux valgus: a randomized controlled trial. JAMA 2001;285(19):2474–80.
16. Reina M, Lafuente G, Munuera PV. Effect of custom-made foot orthoses in female hallux valgus after one-year follow up. Prosthet Orthot Int 2013;37(2):113–9.

17. McDonald MG, Stevens DB. Modified Mitchell bunionectomy for management of adolescent hallux valgus. Clin Orthop Relat Res 1996;(332):163–9.
18. Coughlin MJ. Roger A. Mann Award. Juvenile hallux valgus: etiology and treatment. Foot Ankle Int 1995;16(11):682–97.

Metatarsalgia, Lesser Toe Deformities, and Associated Disorders of the Forefoot

John A. DiPreta, MD

KEYWORDS

- Metatarsalgia • Hammertoe • Metatarsophalangeal joint instability • Gastrocsoleus
- Morton neuroma

KEY POINTS

- Metatarsalgia is a symptom complex of pain localized to the forefoot.
- There are many etiologies to metatarsalgia.
- Hammer toe, mallet toe and claw toe are lesser toe deformities created by an imbalance between the extrinsic and intrinsic musculature of the foot.
- Most conditions of the forefoot can be treated successfully with shoe modifications and off the shelf appliances to alleviate areas of pressure.
- When conservative treatment is unsuccessful, referral to a foot and ankle specialist is necessary to assist the patient in the appropriate selection of corrective procedures.

METATARSALGIA

Metatarsalgia is a term attributed to pain localized to the forefoot region. While there are many conditions that create pain in the forefoot, the term metatarsalgia serves to differentiate such conditions from pain in the area under the second, third, and fourth metatarsal heads.[1]

Pain localized to the forefoot may be associated with disorders of the hallux and lesser toes. It is also important to recognize that in addition to these entities there are conditions of the hindfoot, ankle, and leg that also contribute to metatarsalgia. Distinguishing between these variables can be accomplished through a thorough physical examination.

Classification

Espinosa and colleagues[1] described 3 types of metatarsalgia: primary, secondary, and iatrogenic. Categorization of these entities is useful to help identify the cause of forefoot pain and thus guide treatment.

Division of Orthopaedic Surgery, Albany Medical Center, Albany Medical College, Capital Region Orthopaedics, 1367 Washington Avenue, Suite 200, Albany, NY 12206, USA
E-mail address: jamddipreta@netscape.net

Med Clin N Am 98 (2014) 233–251
http://dx.doi.org/10.1016/j.mcna.2013.10.003
0025-7125/14/$ – see front matter © 2014 Elsevier Inc. All rights reserved.

Primary metatarsalgia is caused by intrinsic abnormalities of metatarsal anatomy and the relationship between the metatarsals and the rest of the foot. The end result is overload to the forefoot. The most common cause is a long second metatarsal.[2] Excess plantarflexion of the forefoot caused by a cavus foot or as a result of a fracture or surgical procedure are additional examples of primary metatarsalgia.[3]

Individuals with large bunion deformities (hallux valgus) may complain of pain in the forefoot caused by incompetence of the first ray (great toe and first metatarsal) in its weight-bearing function, creating transfer pressure to the lesser metatarsals. In addition, primary metatarsalgia can be seen as a consequence of congenital deformities or a neoplastic process that causes enlargement of the metatarsal head.

Individuals with metatarsalgia will experience pain during the midstance phase of gait, which occurs as the foot moves from heel strike to toe off. It is during this phase that the foot makes full contact with the ground. Disorders of the leg, such as contracture of the Achilles tendon complex and leg length discrepancy, can contribute to this type of forefoot pain.[4]

Secondary metatarsalgia can occur as a result of trauma. Fractures of the foot that cause angular or rotational displacement of the metatarsals, resulting in malalignment, may lead to forefoot pain. Additional causes include hallux rigidus (degenerative disease of the hallux metatarsophalangeal [MTP] joint), inflammatory arthropathy, instability of the lesser MTP joints, interdigital neuritis, tarsal tunnel syndrome, and Freiberg infraction.[5] Although these conditions may not exert a direct effect on the metatarsals, they can lead to overload of the forefoot. In addition to trauma affecting metatarsal alignment, damage to the supporting structures of the MTP joint (plantar plate, collateral ligaments) can occur. Injury to these stabilizing structures as a result of a traumatic event or because of inflammatory arthropathy (rheumatoid arthritis) can lead to imbalance of the relationship of the lesser toes to the metatarsal head. This incompetence in the supporting soft tissues around the MTP joint leads to instability and forefoot pain.[6]

Iatrogenic metatarsalgia, as the name implies, may arise as a result of a reconstructive procedure on the foot to address lesser toe abnormality from hallux valgus surgery that has created a shift in plantar pressures to the forefoot.[7] When assessing a patient who complains of forefoot pain, it is important to ask about previous surgical procedures on the foot.

As noted earlier, foot position during the gait cycle will lend clues to the cause of forefoot pain. The gait cycle consists of two components: swing phase and stance phase. Forty percent of the gait cycle is the swing phase with the remaining 60% spent in the stance phase. The stance may be staged simply by 3 time intervals: heel strike, foot flat, and toe off. Pain felt during these intervals can again lend clues to the cause of the pain (**Fig. 1**).

Metatarsalgia felt during heel strike can be seen in the setting of a cavus foot, congenital deformity, or a tight heel cord. Symptoms exhibited during midstance or foot flat are influenced by ankle motion and, therefore, conditions affecting the ankle (degenerative joint disease) may limit dorsiflexion of the ankle and cause pain in the forefoot. During the toe-off phase only the forefoot is in contact with the ground and MTP joints are in a dorsiflexed position. Hammertoes or conditions that create MTP joint instability will be most symptomatic during this phase. It is during this portion of the gait cycle when metatarsalgia occurs most frequently.[1]

Clinical Assessment

As with any encounter with a patient, a thorough history and physical examination is essential. It is important to take note of a history of previous trauma or surgery, as this may change the morphology of the foot. History of diabetes and, in particular,

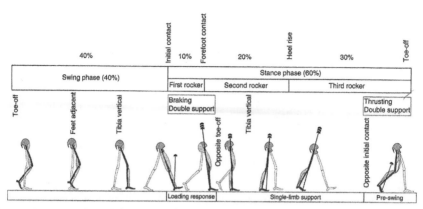

Fig. 1. The gait cycle and the temporal relationships of metatarsalgia and forefoot contact. (©2010 American Academy of Orthopaedic Surgeons. Reprinted from Espinosa N, Brodsky J, Maceira E. Metatarsalgia. J Am Acad Orthop Surg 2010;18:475; with permission.)

diabetic neuropathy is important, as the foot of the diabetic patient may be subject to high forefoot pressures. High forefoot pressure, as seen with a contracture of the gastrocsoleus complex or resulting from lesser toe deformity in combination with neuropathy, can lead to ulceration.

The examination consists of observation of gait and any obvious deformities. A leg-length discrepancy will be associated with a plantarflexion or equinus deformity at the ankle. The patient is examined in the seated and standing position. Assessment of foot shape and associated deformities (hallux valgus, long lesser toes) is documented. It is often helpful to have the patient point to the area of maximal tenderness. Inspection of the foot for ulcerations and/or calluses under the metatarsal heads is performed. Calluses or keratosis may be localized under a particular metatarsal or may be more diffuse in nature. In addition to visual inspection, a neurovascular examination is performed.

Range of motion of the ankle and hindfoot is documented. Ankle stiffness, as seen with degenerative joint disease or an Achilles contracture, should be noted. Passive dorsiflexion that does not go past neutral may be associated with these entities. Assessment of the gastrocsoleus tightness is done by performing the Silfverskiold test. Ankle dorsiflexion is assessed with the knee in full extension and at 90° of knee flexion. The foot is held in an inverted position to avoid motion through the hindfoot. If there is more dorsiflexion with the knee flexed, there is tightness in the gastrocsoleus complex (**Fig. 2**).

Areas of keratosis or plantar callosities should be palpated for tenderness. Inspection of the toes is also performed, documenting the presence of swelling, contracture, and abnormal positioning. Synovitis of the MTP joints (see later discussion) is often a cause of forefoot pain. Swelling of the toe at the level of the MTP joint is a clue to this diagnosis. Along with swelling, deviation of the toe may be seen. One can examine the stability of the MTP joint. The examiner holds the foot with one hand while grasping the toe with the other. The toe is then translated in a dorsal direction (**Fig. 3**). If pain is generated from this maneuver and reproduces the patient's pain, synovitis is suspected.

Palpation of the web space between the metatarsal heads is also recommended. Pain elicited with this maneuver indicates interdigital neuritis (Morton neuroma). The examiner holds the foot with one hand and with the opposite hand squeezes the space

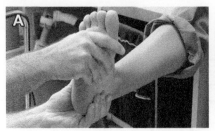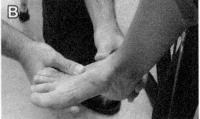

Fig. 2. The Silfverskiold test to assess gastrocsoleus tightness, demonstrating the examination with the knee extended (*A*) and the knee flexed (*B*).

between the metatarsal heads (**Fig. 4**). This action is combined with compression of the forefoot, perhaps inducing a palpable click (Mulder click). Pain elicited is suggestive of interdigital neuritis.

It should also be noted that the forefoot plantar fat pad atrophies with age. With the loss of subcutaneous tissue beneath the metatarsal heads, more pressure is distributed to the bony elements (**Fig. 5**).

Radiologic Examination

Weight-bearing views of the foot in the anteroposterior (AP), lateral, and, in certain cases, oblique projection are necessary. Weight-bearing radiographs of the ankle may also be indicated when ankle abnormality is suspected. The length and inclination of the metatarsals should be assessed. The presence of hallux rigidus or hallux valgus should be noted (**Fig. 6**). The coexistence of these conditions is common with metatarsalgia, and this must be factored into the treatment plan. Additional higher-level imaging (magnetic resonance imaging [MRI] or bone scan) is not routinely indicated.

Treatment

As with any condition, management is guided toward the cause. Symptomatic relief can be achieved with physical therapy, shoe modifications, debridement of calluses, and judicious use of corticosteroid injections.

When gastrocsoleus tightness is contributing to metatarsalgia, a stretching program to lengthen the muscles can be instituted. An effective program is thought to lessen

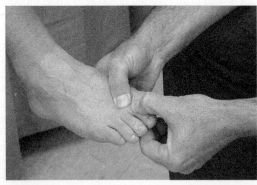

Fig. 3. The dorsal translation test of the second metatarsophalangeal (MTP) joint to assess instability of MTP joint.

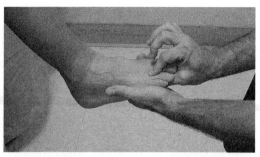

Fig. 4. Palpation of the web space with forefoot compression to evaluate for pathologic symptoms in the interdigital nerve.

the pressure on the forefoot. This program may be best accomplished under the supervision of a physical therapist.[8] A recent study demonstrated the effectiveness of such a regimen by showing an increase in the maximal dorsiflexion and passive tendon length.[9]

The goal of shoe modifications is to dissipate pressure off the forefoot region and to offload specific areas of tenderness. An extra-depth, wide-box shoe can accommodate deformities of the lesser toes, and adding a soft insert can provide additional cushioning. Metatarsal pads and metatarsal bars reduce pressure on the metatarsal head. Custom-made inserts made of accommodative foam material can reduce areas of high plantar pressure.

Judicial use of corticosteroids may be a useful adjunct to the treatment and assessment of metatarsalgia. Injection into the web space for the treatment of interdigital neuritis can provide relief and can differentiate neuritis from other causes of forefoot

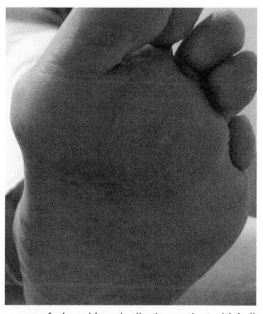

Fig. 5. Clinical appearance of a broad-based callus in a patient with hallux valgus deformity and long lesser metatarsals.

A **B**

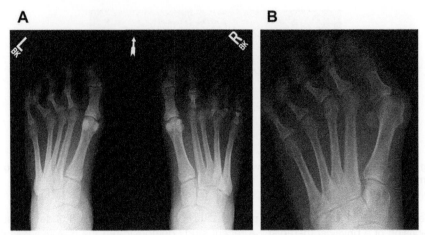

Fig. 6. (*A, B*) Weight-bearing anteroposterior (AP) radiograph of feet demonstrating long metatarsals and instability of lesser MTP joints. Note the dislocation of the third MTP joint on the right foot. Patient with long metatarsals and hallux valgus deformity.

pain. Injections to the MTP joint, while providing relief, carry the risk of causing worsening instability, subluxation, or dislocation. Injection to the soft tissues can lead to fat-pad atrophy.

Paring down the calluses associated with painful keratosis can be helpful in alleviating pain, and can be achieved with a scalpel, callus blade, nail file, or pumice stone. In the short term this can provide symptomatic relief (**Fig. 7**).

Long-term treatment is focused on the underlying cause of metatarsalgia.[6] When conservative measures have been ineffective, referral to a foot and ankle specialist is warranted.

LESSER TOE DEFORMITIES

Lesser toe deformities can create a considerable amount of pain for an individual and negatively affect one's quality of life.[10] Deformities of the forefoot can have multiple causes, which may include a traumatic event, improper shoe wear, neuromuscular disorders, and inflammatory and metabolic diseases. These conditions lead to alterations in the normal anatomy, which ultimately create an imbalance in the muscle-tendon units that control the positioning of the lesser toes.

When the foot is placed into a narrow-box shoe the toes must conform to its shape, which invariably leads to buckling of the toes.[11] With prolonged exposure, flexible deformities can become rigid.

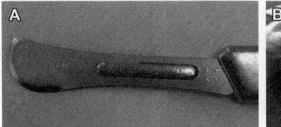 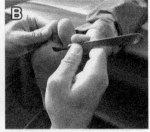

Fig. 7. (*A*) A #17 blade. (*B*) Demonstration of paring of callus with a #17 blade.

Anatomy

To understand the pathologic changes that occur, it is important to understand the anatomy that controls the alignment and position of the lesser toes.

The skeletal anatomy of a lesser toe includes the metatarsal head, the MTP joint, and the proximal, middle, and distal phalanges. The proximal, middle, and distal phalanges are joined at the interphalangeal (IP) joint. Deformity can occur alone or in combination at the IP or MTP joints. The magnitude and direction of the deformity will define the clinical pathology and guide the treatment.

The MTP and IP joints are stabilized by collateral ligaments, joint capsule, and a plantar plate.[12] In addition to these static stabilizers, the dynamic stabilizers of the lesser toes include the extensor digitorum longus (EDL), the extensor digitorum brevis (EDB), and the flexor digitorum longus (FDL) tendons. These tendons are collectively referred to as the extrinsic muscle, as they originate from the lower leg. Their function is to extend the MTP joints and flex the IP joints.

In addition to the extrinsic musculature, the positioning of the lesser toes is affected by the intrinsic muscles, which originate from the bony and soft-tissue elements distal to the forefoot and include the flexor digitorum brevis (FDB), lumbrical muscle, and interosseous muscle. Their purpose is to flex the MTP joints and extend the IP joints (**Fig. 8**).

The position of the toes is maintained by a balance between the stronger extrinsic and weaker intrinsic muscles. Pathologic changes at the MTP joint are created by an imbalance of the static (ligamentous) and dynamic (muscle) stabilizers. With normal walking, the MTP joint dorsiflexes at the heel-rise phase of gait. With hyperextension of the MTP joint, the intrinsics become less efficient as plantarflexors. This deformity progresses as the opposition to the extensors lessen. At the level of the IP joints, the extrinsics (flexors) overpower the weaker intrinsics (extensors). The combination of these pathologic changes leads to a hyperextension deformity at the MTP joint level and a flexion deformity at the IP joint level, creating what is described as a claw toe.[13]

Pathologic Anatomy

The common clinical entities encountered by the primary care physician include hammertoe, mallet toe, and claw toe. These descriptions pertain to the location of the deformity in the toe. Identification of the deformity gives clues to their etiology.

Mallet Toe

Mallet toe is defined by a flexion deformity at the distal interphalangeal (DIP) joint. The proximal interphalangeal (PIP) joint and the MTP joints are in a neutral position (**Fig. 9**A).

Though typically associated with tight shoewear, the specific cause of mallet toe is yet to be defined. The high incidence of mallet toe in women suggests constrictive shoewear as a cause. Constriction of the forefoot causes pressure on the end of the toe, which can ultimately lead to tightness in the FDL tendon. Other causes include inflammatory arthritis, trauma, or a sequela of hammertoe repair.[14] Mallet toe is most commonly seen in the second, third, and fourth toes.

Hammertoe

The hammertoe deformity is characterized by a flexion deformity at the PIP joint with extension at the DIP joint and a neutral or extended position of the MTP joint.[15]

The incidence of hammertoes is seen with constricting shoewear and an aging population.[16] Hammertoes also occur in association with other foot deformities such as

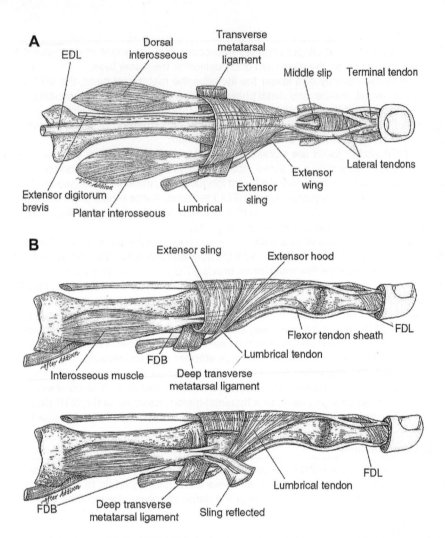

Fig. 8. (*A*, *B*) The tendon, ligament, and bony anatomy of the lesser rays. EDL, extensor digitorum longus; FDB, flexor digitorum brevis; FDL, flexor digitorum longus. (©2011 American Academy of Orthopaedic Surgeons. Reprinted from Shirzad K, Kiesau CD, DeOrio JK, et al. Lesser toe deformities. J Am Acad Orthop Surg 2011;19:505–14; with permission.)

hallux valgus and a long metatarsal. Identification of these entities is essential when formulating a treatment plan (see **Fig. 9**B).

When caused by muscular imbalance, hammertoe deformities may be associated with neuromuscular diseases. Examples include Charcot-Marie-Tooth disease, Friedrich ataxia, myelodysplasia, diabetes mellitus, and Hansen disease.[17] Inflammatory arthropathies such as rheumatoid arthritis and psoriatic arthritis have been implicated with hammertoe deformities.[18]

Claw Toe

The claw-toe is deformity is defined by flexion of both the PIP and DIP joints and hyperextension of the MTP joint (see **Fig. 9**C). It is considered more severe than a

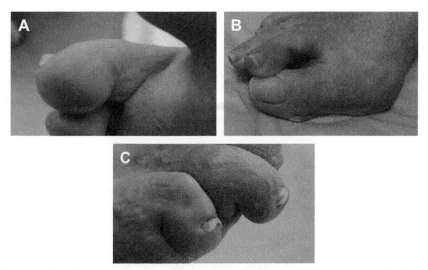

Fig. 9. (*A*) Clinical appearance of a mallet toe. There is a flexion deformity at the distal interphalangeal (DIP) joint. The proximal interphalangeal (PIP) and MTP joints are in a neutral position. (*B*) Clinical appearance of a hammertoe. There is extension of the MTP joint, flexion at the PIP joint, and extension of the DIP joint. It is associated with a hallux valgus deformity. (*C*) Clinical appearance of claw toes in a patient with diabetes mellitus. There is extension of the MTP joint and flexion at the PIP and DIP joints.

hammertoe. As with hammertoe deformities, there is an association with neuromuscular, traumatic, and inflammatory disorders. The claw toe represents an imbalance between the intrinsic and extrinsic muscle units controlling the positioning of the toe.[19] Contracture of the long flexors and extensors without opposition by the foot intrinsics allows the deformity to progress.

Claw toes commonly involve multiple toes and both feet.[20] Other associations include a cavus foot and tight heel cord. The physical deformity leads to the development of painful callosities with shoewear. Callus can develop at the IP joints or plantarly owing to the dorsal subluxation deformity at the MTP joint. As the toe migrates dorsally, the plantar fat pad migrates distally, increasing the prominence of the metatarsal head. In insensate individuals there is a risk for ulceration. A patient may present for an evaluation of the ulcer as the primary complaint.

History and Physical

Patients will present with complaints of pain and difficulty with shoewear, or may have concerns about the appearance of the toe or the presence of callus. Details regarding shoewear problems and a history of trauma or surgery should be noted. A history of diabetes and peripheral neuropathy is important to note, as these deformities put such individuals at significant risk for ulceration.

Examination includes a neurovascular assessment. The presence of diminished or absent sensation would suggest a peripheral neuropathy, prompting further investigation as to whether this represents diabetic peripheral neuropathy or is a result of other systemic illness.

Inspection of the foot should include an assessment of the alignment of the toes while making note of the presence of swelling. The presence of callosities and ulcerations should be documented. These lesions may be seen at the tip of the toe (mallet toe), on the dorsum of the toe at the PIP joint (hammertoe, claw toe), or under one or more metatarsal heads. In long-standing cases, deformities of the toenails can also be seen.

It is important to assess the flexibility of these deformities. If the toe cannot be passively straightened to neutral at the MTP or IP joints, the deformity is considered a rigid deformity. This observation is important, as it helps direct the treatment and education of the patient. Palpation of the MTP and IP joints is necessary to assess for tenderness. Palpation of the web space is important in inspecting for signs of interdigital neuritis, as this too may be a source of forefoot pain.

Radiographic Examination

Radiographs of the affected foot should be obtained in the weight-bearing position if possible. Radiographs are useful to help identify the location and severity of the deformity. AP radiographs will demonstrate the presence and magnitude of lesser metatarsal abnormality, such as a long metatarsal and hallux valgus. Overlap of the proximal phalanx on the metatarsal indicates dislocation of an MTP joint. Presence of arthritic changes at the MTP joint should be noted. Degenerative changes seen at the MTP joint may indicate the presence of Freiberg infraction (avascular necrosis) of the metatarsal head, or erosions (inflammatory arthritis). Lateral radiographs are useful in determining the presence of MTP dislocation and the magnitude of contracture at the IP joints.

Treatment

A trial of conservative measures can be successful as the initial course of treatment. The common goal for these deformities is to relieve pressure from areas of prominence.

Mallet-toe deformities can be treated with the use of commercially available toe sleeves or toe crests (**Fig. 10**). These devices are designed to cushion the tip of the toe, and elevate the toe to alleviate pressure on the tip of the toe (**Fig. 11**). Placement of a soft pad under the foot can soften the contact surface within the shoe. Callus trimming can also be effective. Shoes with a deep toe box and a low heel help reduce the pressure on the tip of the toe.

The approach to hammertoe and claw-toe deformities is similar, with the goal of alleviating pressure on the affected areas. Shoes with a wide toe box and soft uppers will accommodate these deformities. Cutouts made of foam can alleviate pressure at the PIP joint. Gel sleeves are helpful with flexible deformities (**Fig. 12**). When rigid deformities are present, or if there is involvement of the MTP joints, use of metatarsal pads can offload the metatarsal head (**Fig. 13**). A Budin splint can be used to pull the toe down to reduce the PIP-flexion deformity and stabilize the MTP joint, allowing the toe to rest in a more neutral position. Taping around the base of the proximal phalanx to reduce the toe to a neutral position is also an effective tool (**Fig. 14**). When these measures fail to alleviate symptoms and when they are associated with additional foot disorder, an orthosis with an appropriate relief and support can be useful.

Surgical Management

Surgical correction is reserved for failure of conservative treatment and symptoms that persist beyond 6 months. In select individuals with recurrent ulceration, correction is indicated to prevent future ulcerations. Treatment is targeted at correcting the underlying and associated deformities. Correction often requires soft-tissue procedures such as tendon release, transfer or lengthening, or capsular release. Bony procedures

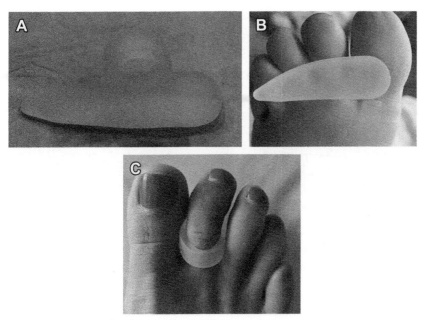

Fig. 10. (*A*) A toe crest. (*B, C*) Example of clinical use of the toe crest.

require joint-resection arthroplasty or implant arthroplasty at the IP joints to correct the fixed flexion deformity. Osteotomies of the metatarsals may also be required to address a long metatarsal or MTP dislocation. Referral to a foot and ankle specialist is most appropriate for surgical consultation (**Fig. 15**).

ASSOCIATED FOREFOOT DEFORMITIES

In addition to the aforementioned lesser toe deformities, 2 additional conditions can be considered along a continuum of progression of lesser toe abnormality: monarticular nontraumatic synovitis and instability, subluxation, and dislocation of the MTP joint.

Monarticular synovitis is characterized by swelling of an isolated MTP joint, which can be seen in the absence of a traumatic event or inflammatory disease.[21] The etiology is thought be related to proliferation of inflammatory synovium. With progression, synovial thickening occurs, leading to distention and stretching of the joint capsule. In

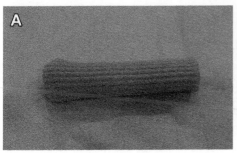
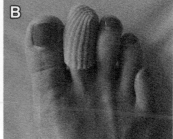

Fig. 11. A closed toe sleeve (*A*) and its clinical use (*B*).

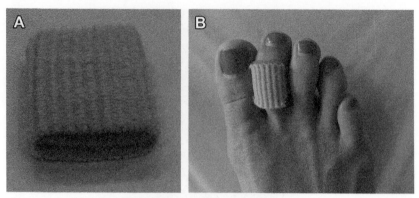

Fig. 12. An open toe sleeve (*A*) and its clinical use (*B*).

turn, this leads to loss of the capsular stabilizing function. The edema within the joint creates a distention force, which clinically manifests as pain. The affected MTP joint will appear swollen and have palpable fullness. It will also feel warm and tender to touch. Range of motion of the involved MTP joint is restricted and is painful. The dorsal drawer test (see **Fig. 3**) may reveal laxity and elicit pain. To perform this test, the examiner grabs the forefoot with one hand and the affected toe with the other. The toe is grasped at the proximal phalanx, and a dorsal translational maneuver is performed. If it creates pain, this test is consistent with monarticular synovitis.

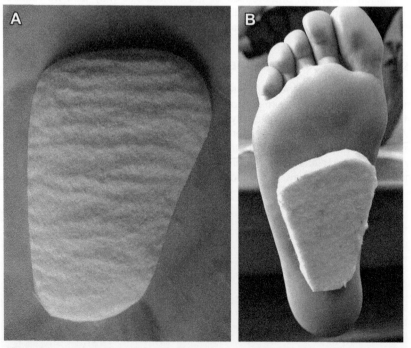

Fig. 13. A metatarsal pad (*A*) and example of its clinical use (*B*). The pad should be placed proximal to the metatarsal heads.

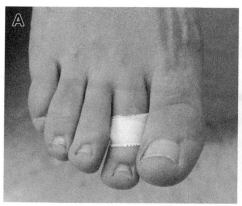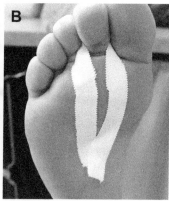

Fig. 14. Clinical example of taping techniques to control position of lesser toe affected by synovitis. (*A*) Dorsal view. (*B*) Plantar view.

Radiographs in the AP projection may reveal widening of the MTP joint. In cases of subluxation, the proximal phalanx may appear in an overlapped position on the metatarsal head. The presence of erosions indicates polyarticular disease.

Treatment consists of shoe modifications, appliances, nonsteroidal anti-inflammatory drugs, and activity restrictions. Shoes with metatarsal supports can

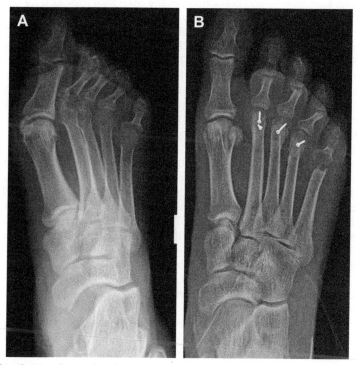

Fig. 15. (*A, B*) AP radiographs of a patient who underwent reconstruction of lesser metatarsal abnormality with soft-tissue and bony repair. The screws demonstrate sites of fixation for metatarsal osteotomies. The fifth metatarsal head was resected.

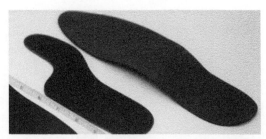

Fig. 16. Carbon-fiber foot plates. These plates allow stiffening of the sole of the shoe. The device on the right would be selectively used for disorders of the great toe, minimizing motion of the first MTP joint.

offload the MTP joint. The use of a carbon-fiber foot plate (**Fig. 16**) can be an effective means to stiffen the sole of the shoe and limit motion across the MTP joints. Corticosteroid injection can be helpful when shoe modifications and other restrictions are unsuccessful. Mizel and Trepman[22] demonstrated success with corticosteroid injection and a stiff-soled shoe for recalcitrant monarticular arthritis. Injections must be administered with caution, as multiple injections or an errantly placed needle may lead to worsening instability.

Surgery is reserved for failure of conservative treatment. Synovectomy, alone or in combination with correction of associated deformities, may be necessary.

Instability, subluxation, and dislocation of the MTP joint may also be seen along this continuum of lesser toe abnormality. Instability may occur as a result of the loss or incompetence of the static stabilizers (joint capsule, collateral ligaments, plantar plate) of the MTP joint. The etiology and pathophysiology are similar to those seen in monarticular synovitis. The clinical appearance is also similar, with warmth and bogginess seen at the MTP joint. As with monarticular synovitis, events during the gait cycle may contribute to deformity. During the toe-off phase the MTP joint dorsiflexes, and with repetitive cycling the plantar plate and capsule elongate. This process can lead to irreversible deformity, which is then compounded by the dynamic imbalance between the intrinsic and extrinsic musculature.

Physical assessment follows that described for lesser toe deformities and monarticular synovitis. Instability assessed with the dorsal drawer test can be appreciated in the affected MTP joint, and comparison is made using the neighboring MTP joints as a control. With progressive deformity, the proximal phalanx moves into greater dorsiflexion and rests on the metatarsal neck. The metatarsal head displaces plantarward and the fat pad moves distally. Because of this functional loss of padding, callosity can form under the metatarsal head.

Radiographic assessment is helpful in assessing the magnitude of the deformity, and may give clues to the diagnosis. The same techniques as in the assessment of lesser toe abnormality are used. The presence of associated (hallux valgus, long metatarsal) deformities can also be evaluated.

Treatment is targeted at symptomatic relief through the use of an extra-depth shoe, metatarsal pads, and soft inserts. Rocker-bottomed shoes to offload the metatarsal heads may also prove useful. When conservative measures fail to provide symptomatic relief, surgery is indicated. The surgical approach would also include synovectomy as described for monarticular synovitis; however, the presence and magnitude of the deformity at the MTP joint must be assessed and the appropriate correction selected. When other deformities coexist, correction of these may also need to be incorporated into the treatment plan.

DISORDERS OF THE PLANTAR SKIN

Discrete intractable plantar keratoses and diffuse plantar keratoses are conditions of the plantar skin associated with hyperkeratotic disorders of the skin. A discrete plantar keratosis is typically seen under a singular metatarsal head, and can be a significant source of pain and disability.[23] These "seed corns" are characterized by a core of avascular tissue that is tender to direct pressure. It is typically localized under a metatarsal head, and may be associated with a prominent fibular condyle (**Fig. 17**). Radiographs, when obtained with a lead marker over the lesion, may help localize the underlying disorder.

Office-based management includes recommendations for the use of metatarsal pads and soft-soled inserts. Metatarsal pads are placed proximal to the metatarsal head to offload that region of the forefoot. Shaving of the callus can also be performed periodically in the office. Maintenance can be achieved through the use of a pumice stone on the affected areas after bathing.

Surgical intervention for these lesions is aimed at the underlying cause. It typically will require removing a bony prominence formed by the plantar condyles of the metatarsal head.

Diffuse plantar keratoses are typically broader based. Their presence under the metatarsal heads is due to abnormal pressure. This increased pressure may be a manifestation of a short first metatarsal or functionally long lesser metatarsals, and can also be seen as a sequela of a traumatic event that alters the weight-bearing function of the first ray, causing transfer metatarsalgia. Fractures of the lesser metatarsals can create these lesions when the fractures heal in a plantarflexed position.

Management is aimed at offloading of the areas of pressure. Options for this include the use of pads, custom orthoses, and/or soft inserts. Surgery is reserved for recalcitrant cases, and requires careful assessment of the underlying cause and radiographic studies to determine the appropriate correction. The goal of surgery is to restore more normal mechanical alignment and balance across the forefoot. Referral to a foot and ankle specialist is necessary in these cases and when there has been a history of trauma, or in an individual at high risk for complications, such as a patient with diabetes mellitus and peripheral neuropathy.

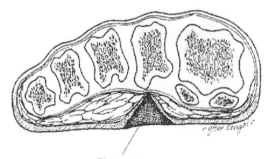

Plantar keratosis

Fig. 17. Anatomy of a prominent metatarsal condyle creating a plantar keratosis. (©1995 American Academy of Orthopaedic Surgeons. Reprinted from Mizel M, Yodlowksi ML. Disorders of the lesser metatarsophalangeal joints. J Am Acad Orthop Surg 1995;3:166–73; with permission.)

INTERDIGITAL NEURALGIA (MORTON NEUROMA)

Interdigital neuralgia (IDN) is also a common form of forefoot pain, commonly referred to as Morton neuroma. Morton described an affliction of the fourth MTP joint and the lateral plantar nerve and its treatment, which included methods of surgical resection, blood letting, and anodyne treatment.[24] Common descriptions are inaccurate in that it does not represent a nerve tumor.[25]

Etiology, Anatomy, and Pathophysiology

The term neuralgia may most accurately describe the clinical presentation of this condition coupled with absence of inflammatory changes in the nerve and surrounding structures on histologic examination.[26] The interdigital nerves (branches of the posterior tibial nerve) travel on the plantar surface of the foot, emerge plantar to the transverse metatarsal ligament (TML), and bifurcate to provide sensation to the adjacent toes (**Fig. 18**). Variations in the anatomy of the forefoot may contribute to the development of symptoms, but the exact cause is unknown. These variations may include spacing of the metatarsal heads, alteration in TML orientation after forefoot trauma, and mobility of the surrounding metatarsals. A direct injury to the nerve by a penetrating wound or crush injury may lead to a painful neuroma and clinical symptoms. Overuse, or repetitive microtrauma in dancers, runners, or other athletes who participate in sports, creating high forefoot forces, may also be at risk.[26]

History and Physical Examination

A patient will typically describe pain in the forefoot in between the metatarsal heads, and may also describe a feeling of fullness or "walking on a pebble." The quality of pain

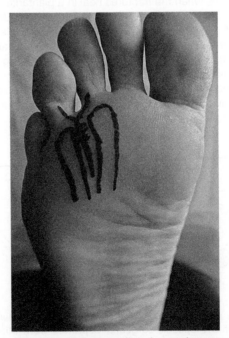

Fig. 18. Trace depicting the course of the interdigital nerve between the metatarsal heads, underneath the transverse metatarsal ligament.

is typically sharp, tingling, or burning in nature, and radiates into the toes. The symptoms are typically unilateral and are localized to a single web space. The third web space is the most commonly involved, although the second web space may also be involved. IDN involving the first and fourth web spaces is rare.

Symptoms are exacerbated by tight-fitting shoes, such as dress or high-heeled shoes. A patient may describe relief by rubbing the foot. It is important to evaluate the patient's shoewear. It is useful to trace out the person's foot on a piece of paper and place the shoe over the tracing to demonstrate the discrepancy between the shoe size and the foot.[27]

The physical examination should include inspection for deformities of the toes, evidence of callus formation, and areas of swelling or bruising. Examination should be performed with the patient seated and standing. One must also inspect the MTP joints for evidence of instability, as this may mimic symptoms associated with IDN. Plantar palpation of the web spaces will elicit pain in the patient. Forefoot compression with palpation of the web space may elicit a "clunk" and the patient's symptoms (see **Fig. 4**).

Radiographic Studies

Weight-bearing radiographs of the foot in the AP, oblique, and lateral projections are used to evaluate osseous deformities. One should make note of the presence of subluxation or dislocation of the MTP joints or evidence of metatarsal fractures. The use of advanced imaging is typically not necessary, as ultrasonography and MRI have not been shown to be more accurate than clinical examination alone.[28] Electrodiagnostic studies are not necessary to make the diagnosis unless one suspects a lumbar radiculopathy.

Treatment

Treatment initially is focused on shoewear modification, consisting of a wider-boxed shoe with a soft insert. Use of a metatarsal pad or neuroma pad placed proximal to the lesion can also be helpful. If IDN is associated with other forefoot symptoms (MTP synovitis), a rocker-bottom shoe or modification with a metatarsal bar may also prove beneficial.

Corticosteroid injection may also be offered as a diagnostic and a therapeutic tool. The volume injected should not exceed 1.5 mL, as greater volumes can potentially cause damage to adjacent structure (tendon, joint capsules). Greenfield and colleagues[29] demonstrated improvement in 60% to 80% of those treated with injection; however at 2 years only 30% showed continued benefit.

The use of alcohol solutions has also been described for the treatment of IDN. Results of multiple injections may be useful in reducing pain in up 89% of patients.[30] Other pharmacologic agents include vitamin B_6, and antidepressant and antiseizure medications.[26]

Nonoperative therapy is effective in most patients, although up to 60% to 70% of patients elect to undergo surgical intervention when symptoms prevail. Individuals may choose to undergo surgery when modifications fail or they are no longer willing to make adjustments to their shoewear or lifestyle. Surgical intervention, when chosen, is resection of the interdigital nerve in the affected web space.

SUMMARY

Forefoot disorders can be a considerable source of pain and dysfunction. Obtaining a careful history and performing a focused examination will help identify the cause of the pain. Once the cause is identified, treatment can be instituted. Treatment with shoe modifications, appliances, and the judicious use of corticosteroids is successful. When conservative measures fail, surgical intervention should be entertained and a referral to a foot and ankle specialist should be made.

REFERENCES

1. Espinosa N, Brodsky J, Maceira E. Metatarsalgia. J Am Acad Orthop Surg 2010; 18:474–85.
2. Maestro M, Besse JL, Ragusa M, et al. Forefoot morphotype study and planning method for forefoot osteotomy. Foot Ankle Clin 2003;8:695–710.
3. Crosbie J, Burns J, Ouvrier RA. Pressure characteristics in painful pes cavus feet resulting from Charcot-Marie-Tooth Disease. Gait Posture 2008;28:545–51.
4. Ledoux WR, Shofer JB, Ahroni JH, et al. Biomechanical differences among pes cavus, neutrally aligned and pes planus feet in subjects with diabetes. Foot Ankle Int 2003;24:845–50.
5. Espinosa N, Maceira E, Myerson MS. Current concept review: metatarsalgia. Foot Ankle Int 2008;29:871–9.
6. Coughlin MJ. Common causes of pain in the forefoot in adults. J Bone Joint Surg Br 2000;82:781–90.
7. Vora AM, Myerson MS. First metatarsal osteotomy non-union and malunion. Foot Ankle Clin 2005;10:35–54.
8. Dockery GL. Evaluation and treatment of metatarsalgia and keratotic disorders. In: Myerson M, editor. Foot and ankle disorders. Philadelphia: Saunders; 2000. p. 359–77.
9. Gazdosik RL, Allred JD, Gabbert HL, et al. A stretching program increases the dynamic passive length and passive resistive properties of calf muscle-tendon unit of unconditioned younger women. Eur J Appl Physiol 2007;99: 449–54.
10. Chen J, Devine A, Dick IM, et al. Prevalence of lower extremity pain, its functionality and quality of life in elderly members in Australia. J Rheumatol 2003;30(12): 2689–93.
11. Coughlin MJ, Dorris J, Polk E. Operative repair of the fixed hammertoe deformity. Foot Ankle Int 2000;21(2):94–104.
12. Sarrafian SK, Topouzian LK. The anatomy and physiology of the extensor apparatus of the toes. J Bone Joint Surg Am 1969;51(4):669–79.
13. Mizel M, Yodlowksi ML. Disorders of the lesser metatarsophalangeal joints. J Am Acad Orthop Surg 1995;3:166–73.
14. Coughlin MJ. Operative repair of the mallet toe deformity. Foot Ankle Int 1995; 16(3):109–16.
15. Coughlin MJ. Lesser toe deformities. In: Coughlin MJ, Mann RA, Saltzman CL, editors. Surgery of the foot and ankle, vol 1, 8th edition. Philadelphia: Mosby Elsevier; 2007. p. 363–464.
16. Coughlin MJ, Thompson FM. The high price of high fashion footwear. Instr Course Lect 1995;44:371–7.
17. Coughlin MJ. Subluxation and dislocation of the second metatarsophalangeal joint. Orthop Clin North Am 1989;20(4):535–51.
18. Coughlin MJ. Mallet toes, hammertoes, claw toes and corns. Causes of lesser toe deformities. Postgrad Med 1984;75(5):191–8.
19. Mills GP. The etiology and treatment of clawfoot. J Bone Joint Surg 1924;6:142–9.
20. Coughlin MJ. Lesser toe abnormalities. J Bone Joint Surg Am 2002;84:1446–69.

21. Mann R, Mizel MS. Monarticular non-traumatic synovitis of the MTP joint. A new diagnosis? Foot Ankle 1985;6:18–21.
22. Mizel MS, Trepman ET. Nonoperative treatment of MTP joint synovitis. Foot Ankle 1993;14:305.
23. Mann RA. Intractable plantar keratoses. Instr Course Lect 1984;33:287–301.
24. Larson EE, Barrett SL, Battiston B, et al. Accurate nomenclature for forefoot nerve entrapment: a historical perspective. J Am Podiatr Med Assoc 2005;95(3): 298–306.
25. Giannini S, Bacchini P, Ceccarelli F, et al. Interdigital neuroma: clinical examination and histopathologic results in 63 cases treated with excision. Foot Ankle Int 2004;25(2):79–84.
26. Peters PG, Adams SB, Schon LC. Interdigital neuralgia. Foot Ankle Clin 2011;16: 305–15.
27. Kay D, Bennett GL. Morton's neuroma. Foot Ankle Clin 2003;8(1):49–59.
28. Sharp RJ, Wade CM, Hennessy MS, et al. The role of MRI and ultrasound imaging in Morton's neuroma and the effect of size of lesion on symptoms. J Bone Joint Surg Br 2003;85(7):999–1005.
29. Greenfield J, Rea J, Ilfeld FW. Morton's interdigital neuroma. Indications for treatment by local injections versus surgery. Clin Orthop Relat Res 1984;(185):142–4.
30. Dockery GL. The treatment of intermetatarsal neuromas with 4% alcohol sclerosing injections. J Foot Ankle Surg 1999;38(6):403–8.

Arthritides of the Foot

Samuel G. Dellenbaugh, MD[a],*, Jorge Bustillo, MD[b]

KEYWORDS

- Midfoot arthritis • Hallux rigidus • Hindfoot arthritis • Arthrodesis

KEY POINTS

- Arthritis of the first metatarsophalangeal joint is the most common arthritis of the foot.
- Midfoot arthritis is commonly due to traumatic events whereas hindfoot arthritis can be due to trauma or deformity.
- Initial treatment of foot arthritis starts with symptomatic treatment and orthotics.
- Surgical treatment of foot arthritis is typically through arthrodesis.

INTRODUCTION

Arthritis is becoming more of a problem with the aging of the population. By 2030, 72.1 million people will be older than 65 years in the United States, more than doubling since 2000.[1] As people get older, the incidence of arthritis increases; people with arthritis have a significantly lower physical and mental quality of life, with more than twice as many people reporting fair or poor health as compared with people without arthritis.[2] The increasing incidence of arthritis as the US population gets older makes this an important problem for doctors to treat.

Arthritis in the foot can be broken down into 3 subgroups. The first metatarsophalangeal joint can become arthritic in a disease process known as *hallux rigidus*. Second, the tarsometatarsal joints can degenerate, most commonly secondary to an inciting traumatic event. And third, the joints around the hindfoot can become arthritic, either caused by trauma or deformity. These 3 subgroups are discussed in turn through the course of this article.

HALLUX RIGIDUS

The term *hallux rigidus* (Latin for "stiff toe") is used to describe the symptoms of degenerative arthritis of the first metatarsophalangeal joint. Initially described by Davies-Colley[3] in 1887, the term *hallux rigidus* was then coined by Cotterill[4] a few months later. *Hallux limitus* is also used to describe osteoarthritis of the first

[a] OrthoNY, 121 Everett Road, Albany, NY 12205, USA; [b] Penn State Hershey Bone and Joint Institute, 30 Hope Drive, Building B, Suite 2400, Hershey, PA 17033-0850, USA
* Corresponding author.
E-mail address: sdellenbaugh@gmail.com

Med Clin N Am 98 (2014) 253–265
http://dx.doi.org/10.1016/j.mcna.2013.10.004   **medical.theclinics.com**
0025-7125/14/$ – see front matter © 2014 Elsevier Inc. All rights reserved.

metatarsophalangeal joint, whereas *hallux rigidus* describes the same condition with no range of motion of the joint.[5] This condition has been reported to be present in 2.5% of people older than 50 years, making it the most common arthritic condition of the foot.[6] This condition occurs more commonly in women,[7,8] and two-thirds of patients have some positive family history of the disorder.[9]

PRESENTATION

Patients with hallux rigidus typically present with pain and swelling of the great toe metatarsophalangeal joint. Synovitis of this joint and decreased dorsiflexion is also seen. The degenerative osteoarthritis of the joint typically starts dorsally and dorsolaterally, with noted bony osteophyte formation.[5] These osteophytes abut the dorsal aspect of the proximal phalanx, decreasing dorsiflexion of the metatarsophalangeal joint. A dorsal prominence over the proximal aspect of the metatarsophalangeal joint is typically present and is inflamed and painful because of rubbing against the shoe. The dorsomedial cutaneous branch of the superficial peroneal nerve can also become irritated, and dysesthesias or paresthesias along the medial aspect of the hallux can be present.[7]

Physical examination will show a decreased range of motion of the first metatarsophalangeal joint, especially in dorsiflexion. Pain can be elicited in extremes of dorsiflexion and plantarflexion early in the disease; as the disease progresses, pain will start to show up in the midrange of motion. Patients will complain of increased pain with running and going up on their toes, such as in the toe-off section of the gait. Patients will walk with an antalgic gait, attempting to unload the medial column of the foot and decrease the motion of the arthritic first metatarsophalangeal joint through the gait cycle. This gait will start to overload the lateral column of the foot, causing lateral foot pain.

The initial radiographic evaluation of hallux rigidus should be standing anteroposterior (AP), lateral, and oblique projections. Radiographic classification of hallux rigidus has been described by Coughlin and Shurnas[10] and is shown in **Table 1**. Magnetic resonance imaging (MRI) and computed tomography (CT) evaluation is not required unless an osteochondral lesion was suspected. Osteophytes start to appear in later stages on the metatarsal head and the proximal phalanx. Osteophytes manifest initially on the dorsal aspect of the joint, obscuring the joint space (**Fig. 1**). Cartilage loss starts initially on the dorsal aspect of the joint and progresses plantarly, sometimes expanding to the sesamoids.[9]

Table 1 Grading of hallux rigidus	
Grade 0	Dorsiflexion of 40°–60° (20% loss of motion), normal radiographs and no pain
Grade 1	Dorsiflexion of 30°–40°, dorsal osteophytes, minimal to no other joint changes
Grade 2	Dorsiflexion of 10°–30°, mild flattening of MTP joint, mild to moderate joint space narrowing or sclerosis, osteophytes
Grade 3	Dorsiflexion of less than 10°, decreased plantar flexion, hypertrophied cysts, erosions, or irregular sesamoids on radiograph; moderate to severe pain, pain at extremes of range of motion
Grade 4	Stiff toe, radiographs showing loose bodies or osteochondral defects, pain throughout range of motion

Abbreviation: MTP, metatarsophalangeal.

From Coughlin MJ, Shurnas PS. Hallux rigidus: grading and long-term results of operative treatment. J Bone Joint Surg Am 2003;85(11):2073.

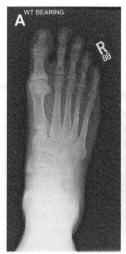

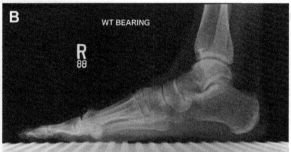

Fig. 1. (A) AP weight-bearing radiograph of the foot showing decreased joint space of the first metatarsophalangeal (MTP) joint, moderate-grade hallux rigidus. (B) Lateral weight-bearing radiograph of the foot showing dorsal osteophyte of the first MTP joint, moderate-grade hallux rigidus. WT, weight.

NONOPERATIVE TREATMENT

Nonoperative treatment should be tried first. Nonsteroidal antiinflammatory drugs can decrease joint swelling and pain but have little prolonged clinical effect. Intraarticular corticosteroid injections can also decrease local swelling and pain but have minimal long-term benefits and can cause articular cartilage damage. Solan and colleagues[11] reported on intraarticular steroid injections, showing that one-third of patients with early (grade 1) disease had pain relief for 6 months before requiring surgery, whereas two-thirds of patients with moderate (grade 2) disease and all patients with severe (grade 3) disease required surgery at a median time of 2 months. Pons and colleagues[12] published a comparison of intraarticular injections of corticosteroids and sodium hyaluronate. Both groups showed significantly reduced pain at the 3-month follow-up. However, approximately half of both groups went on to surgical intervention within 1 year.

Shoe modification can be helpful to decrease dorsiflexion of the metatarsophalangeal joint and, thereby, decrease pain. Stiff shoe inserts, such as a Morton's extension, made of rigid orthotic material decrease this dorsiflexion. A rocker-bottom sole can also decrease dorsiflexion. Wide or high toe box shoes can decrease rubbing of shoes on osteophytes and the commensurate pain. These modifications are often not well tolerated by patients, especially by women.[9]

OPERATIVE TREATMENT

Patients who have failed nonoperative treatment of hallux rigidus often go on to operative treatment. There are a variety of different surgical techniques for the treatment of hallux rigidus, which can be characterized as either joint preserving or joint sacrificing.

Joint-preserving procedures are a series of procedures that do not include fusion of the metatarsophalangeal joint. These procedures address the problematic impingement of the proximal phalanx and the distal metatarsal. In addition, they make some attempt to address the arthritis within the first metatarsophalangeal joint. Joint-preserving procedures include cheilectomy, with or without a proximal phalangectomy; Keller resection osteotomy; interposition arthroplasty; and hemiarthroplasty.

Cheilectomy, first described in 1959 by DuVries,[13] typically consists of the excision of approximately 30% of the dorsal metatarsal head articular surface and the dorsal metaphyseal and phalangeal osteophytes as well as the release of the medial and lateral joint capsule and ligaments. This procedure allows more normal dorsiflexion of the metatarsophalangeal joint, partially decompresses the joint, and retains motion and stability of the joint (**Fig. 2**). In addition, it offers the opportunity to perform further procedures on the toe.[7,14] Consistent results in several studies support the use of cheilectomy in lower-grade (1 and 2) hallux rigidus, with a 92% success rate noted in a 2003 study by Coughlin and Shurnas.[7,10,15] Cheilectomy can be combined with a proximal phalangeal closing wedge osteotomy, as described by Moberg,[16] thus converting a portion of the plantar flexion arc to dorsiflexion. The primary cause of cheilectomy failure is inadequate bone resection. However, with greater than 30% to 40% resection of the metatarsal head, subluxation or avascular necrosis can be seen. In addition, cheilectomies on patients who have pain in the midrange of motion have been shown to have poor intermediate- to long-term results.[17]

The Keller excisional arthroplasty and the interpositional arthroplasty have been postulated to be procedures in the middle ground between cheilectomy and arthrodesis. The Keller excisional arthroplasty, first described in 1904,[18] describes the excision of the base of the proximal phalanx in an effort to decompress the first metatarsophalangeal joint in patients who are elderly or are low demand. However, this has been found to lead to multiple complications, including a floppy great toe, transfer metatarsalgia, and a cock-up deformity of the great toe.[19–21] Patients continue to have motion at the first metatarsophalangeal joint, but the joint has been destabilized. The interpositional arthroplasty has been described by many people[22–25] and is typically a Keller excisional arthroplasty with the subsequent interposition of soft tissue into the metatarsophalangeal joint. This soft tissue can be either allograft or autograft; techniques using the plantaris, gracilis, and/or extensor hallucis brevis tendons or the joint capsule itself have been described. However, the data at this time do not support the use of this technique because the results have been mixed.[7] Replacement of the first metatarsophalangeal joint with either a total or hemiarthroplasty is controversial. Some studies show good early and midterm follow-up results, but results more than 5 years after surgery are unknown. One study by Gibson and Thomson[26] comparing arthrodesis with total joint replacement showed a much higher complication rate in the arthroplasty arm, with the cost of the arthrodesis being half of the arthroplasty. Forty percent of the patients in the study would not undergo arthroplasty again.

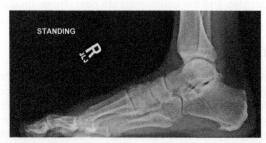

Fig. 2. Lateral radiograph of the foot after first metatarsophalangeal joint cheilectomy.

Arthrodesis of the first metatarsophalangeal joint is the current gold standard for the management of severe (grade 3–4) hallux rigidus (**Fig. 3**). Even though the motion of the first metatarsophalangeal joint is lost, this procedure gives predictable long-term pain relief. Various techniques have been described, but the most important part of the operative procedure is to place the toe into the appropriate position: 10° to 20° of valgus, 10°to 15° of dorsiflexion with respect to the first tarsometatarsal joint, and 20° to 30° of dorsiflexion with regard to the floor (**Fig. 4**). The outcomes of this procedure have been good. Patients have been shown to fuse the joint about 94% of the time.[16] Postoperatively, patients have improvement in propulsive power, function during weight bearing, and stability during gait,[27] albeit with a shorter step length and some loss of ankle plantar flexion at toe-off.[28]

MIDFOOT ARTHRITIS

Arthritis of the midfoot, specifically of the tarsometatarsal joints, can be a debilitating problem affecting 1 in 55,000 people.[29] The common causes include osteoarthritis; inflammatory arthritis, such as rheumatoid arthritis; Charcot neuroarthropathy (most commonly secondary to poorly controlled diabetes); and traumatic injuries, such as a Lisfranc fracture dislocation. Traumatic injuries to the lower extremity have increased with the advent of air bags; a 2007 retrospective study of front-end motor vehicle accidents involving air bag deployment showed that injuries to the foot and ankle were the second most common (38.4%), with only injuries to the hip, thigh, and knee being more common (49.5%).[30]

Anatomic and biomechanical considerations combine to cause the specific presentation of midfoot arthritis. The midfoot is made up of 3 columns. The medial column is made up of the first metatarsal and the medial cuneiform. The middle column is made up of the second and third metatarsals and the intermediate and lateral cuneiforms. The lateral column is made up of the fourth and fifth metatarsals as well as the cuboid. Ligamentous complexes hold these columns together dorsally, plantarly, and in between the cuneiforms; the plantar and intercuneiform are stronger than the dorsal. The navicular bridges the medial and middle columns. The lateral column is the most mobile, with up to 10° of mobility in the sagittal plane. This mobility allows the

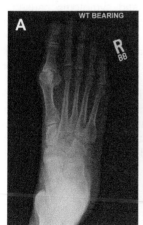
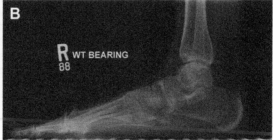

Fig. 3. (*A*) AP weight-bearing radiograph of the foot with high-grade hallux rigidus. (*B*) Lateral weight-bearing radiograph of the foot with high-grade hallux rigidus. WT, weight.

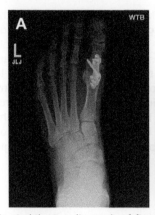
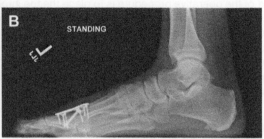

Fig. 4. (*A*) AP radiograph of first metatarsophalangeal (MTP) joint arthrodesis, (*B*) Lateral radiograph of first MTP joint arthrodesis. WTB, weight bearing.

joints to move to the least-painful location; therefore, arthritis in the lateral column is the least symptomatic. The medial and central columns, however, are much less mobile, with the second tarsometatarsal joint being the least mobile. This lack of mobility does not allow the joints to move to the less-symptomatic locations; therefore, arthritis in these joints is more symptomatic. With advanced disease, the biomechanics of the foot are altered because of the instability of the tarsometatarsal joints and the subsequent osteophyte formation, leading to the foot becoming pronated, dorsiflexed through the tarsometatarsal joints, and abducted. In one study, 78% of patients with midfoot arthritis presented with abnormal foot posture or with difficulty in wearing shoes.[31] This deformity through the midfoot leads to a rigid pes planus configuration.

PRESENTATION

Patients with midfoot arthritis typically present with complaints of pain. This pain is a deep aching pain and is worsened with weight bearing. With progression of the disease, pes planus ensues, creating bony prominences both dorsally and plantarly, causing pain. Patients can also have neuritic signs and symptoms caused by compression of the deep peroneal nerve, the superficial peroneal nerve, and the saphenous nerve. The extensor tendons can become inflamed, causing pain with extension of the toes. Patients can also complain of pain with physical examination movements, specifically piano key–like movements of the tarsometatarsal joints and pronation and abduction of the forefoot.

Radiographic evaluation of midfoot arthritis starts with a standard 3-view radiograph series: AP, lateral, and oblique (**Fig. 5**). These radiographs will show any gross abnormalities and help to identify the location and extent of arthritis. Bone scans can be used to look at any areas suspected of infection or stress fractures. CT scans are useful to look at the intricacies of the bony anatomy, and MRI scans may be helpful in early inflammatory arthritis.

NONOPERATIVE TREATMENT

The goal of nonoperative treatment of midfoot arthritis is to decrease motion and instability across the midfoot, decrease pain, and relieve pressure from bony prominences. Nonsteroidal antiinflammatory drugs are an integral part of the treatment of

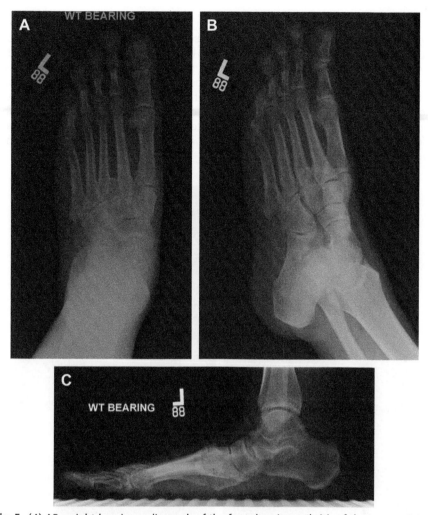

Fig. 5. (*A*) AP weight-bearing radiograph of the foot showing arthritis of the tarsometatar-sal joints. (*B*) Oblique radiograph of the foot with tarsometatarsal arthritis. (*C*) Lateral weight-bearing radiograph of the foot showing midfoot arthritis and subsequent midfoot sag deformity (loss of arch). WT, weight.

any arthritis and are useful in treating midfoot arthritis. These drugs can have some detrimental effects on the gastrointestinal and cardiovascular systems of patients; therefore, extended use is not recommended.[32] Shoe modification and stiff-soled orthoses are often used in the treatment of midfoot arthritis. Stiff-soled shoes and rocker-bottom shoes change transfer weight during the gait cycle by decreasing the time and pressure that the midfoot experiences.[33] This decreases the symptoms of pain and stiffness that continued movement of the midfoot causes and is similar to the stiffening strategy of decreasing the motion of the midfoot seen in kinematic studies of patients with midfoot arthritis.[34] Ankle-foot clamshell orthoses can also be used to restrict the movement of the foot and ankle in order to alleviate symptoms, with a decrease in pressure on the plantar foot of as much as 30%.[35]

OPERATIVE TREATMENT

Surgical treatment of midfoot arthritis can be separated into the treatment of 2 separate areas: the medial/middle column and the lateral column. Instability of the medial and middle columns is typically treated with arthrodesis of the first, second, and third tarsometatarsal joints and the respective intercuneiform joints. This treatment requires restoration of the normal mechanical alignment of the foot, preparation of the joint surfaces through the removal of any remaining cartilage, and rigid stabilization of the joints with either lag screws or screws and plates (**Fig. 6**). This surgery is done through 2 longitudinal incisions, one between the first and second metatarsals and the other over the fourth metatarsal.

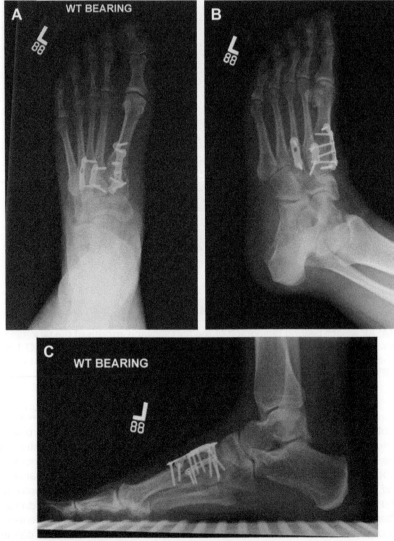

Fig. 6. (*A*) AP radiograph of midfoot arthrodesis. (*B*) Oblique radiograph of midfoot arthrodesis. (*C*) Lateral radiograph of midfoot arthrodesis. WT, weight.

Treatment of arthritis of the lateral column differs from that of the medial column because the lateral column is significantly more mobile than the medial column, and few studies in the literature show that fusion of this more mobile column is successful. It is thought that arthrodesis of these lateral rays can lead to chronic lateral foot pain, nonunion, and an increased risk of stress fracture.[36] Fusion of the lateral column in midfoot arthritis is not strictly contraindicated and may be helpful in patients with lateral midfoot collapse or rocker bottom deformity,[37] but motion-preserving procedures are considered more beneficial. Berlet and colleagues[38] retrospectively looked at the outcomes of patients who had their lateral tarsometatarsal joints resected with the interposition of peroneus tertius in the resultant space. Six of 8 patients who underwent the procedure were satisfied with the surgery; their pain decreased, on average, 35% from preoperative levels. More recently, Shawen and colleagues[39] placed ceramic spheres into the lateral tarsometatarsal joints after they were debrided. This configuration was theorized to maintain the mobility of the lateral column while removing the pain that was generating arthritis. At an average follow-up of 34 months, the group of 13 patients reported that their pain, measured by an analog visual scale, decreased 42% and their American Orthopaedic Foot and Ankle Society scores improved 87%. Both methods have had their own level of success, showing that maintaining mobility of the lateral column of the foot can have success in alleviating pain in lateral midfoot arthritis.

Arthrodesis of the midfoot can be complicated by several problems. Nonunion occurs in approximately 3% to 7% of patients and is highest in elderly patients.[27,28] Second, patients can have pain from retained hardware in approximately 9% of surgeries,[40] and the formation of postoperative neuromas occurs in up to 7% of patients.[41] Long-term complications can include sesamoid pain, likely caused by the increased stiffness of the medial column; metatarsalgia; stress fractures; and exacerbation of adjacent joint arthritis.[40]

HINDFOOT ARTHRITIS

The subtalar joint acts as a mitered hinge, translating motion from the transverse tarsal joint to the tibiotalar joint, by moving through a range of between 15° of eversion and 30° of inversion. During the gait cycle, the subtalar joint moves through its range of motion. As the heel strikes the ground, the inverted subtalar joint rapidly everts, thus, making the talonavicular and calcaneocuboid joints parallel and supple. This allows for maximum energy dissipation at the foot's impact with the ground. Once the foot reaches its maximum eversion, the subtalar joint then begins to invert, thus, causing the talonavicular and calcaneocuboid joints to diverge. This causes the foot to become a rigid lever arm and assists in the propulsive phase of the gait.

Arthritis of the subtalar joint can have multiple causes. Commonly, posttraumatic subtalar arthritis is seen secondary to prior calcaneus or talus fractures. Primary subtalar arthritis is uncommon and usually is caused by residual deformity secondary to tarsal coalition, posterior tibial tendon dysfunction, or instability. Patients with inflammatory arthritis can show symptoms and signs of arthritic degeneration of the subtalar joint.

Regardless of the cause, patients usually present with pain in the lateral hindfoot. This pain is compounded by feelings of instability, catching, or locking and can be aggravated by walking on uneven ground. The hindfoot can swell and feel stiff. Typically, the evaluation of the hindfoot begins with weight-bearing radiographs of the ankle and foot, including AP, oblique, and lateral projections. Specialized views, such as the Broden view, can show the posterior subtalar facet and can be done by rotating the foot internally 45° and then angling the x-ray beam between 10° and 40° cephalad. The Harris axial view is another specialized view that can show the posterior and middle facet joints. This view is achieved by angling the x-ray beam approximately 45° to the horizontal while obtaining an image along the long axis of the calcaneus. More advanced imaging can be useful; the CT scan (**Fig. 7**) is good for visualizing fine details of bony anatomy, and the MRI is good for visualizing soft tissue and non-bony anatomy.

NONOPERATIVE TREATMENT

Nonoperative management for hindfoot arthritis is typically the treatment of symptoms. As in most orthopedic problems, treatment begins with pain control and the use of nonsteroidal antiinflammatory drugs. These drugs can decrease painful symptoms as well as the inflammation associated with the arthritis. Physical therapy is also useful, focusing on increasing the range of motion, muscle strength, and proprioception. Modification of the patients' activity can also improve symptoms. Subtalar injections can be useful to both diagnose the cause of pain and to treat the pain itself.

The modification of footwear and the use of orthotics is an integral part of the treatment of symptomatic hindfoot arthritis. These orthotics and braces limit painful motions and relieve pressure points. They can both be accommodative for rigid deformities and correct flexible ones. Multiple types of braces can be used, including the University of California Berkeley Laboratory insert, the hinged Ankle Foot Orthosis, an air cast, and lace-up ankle braces.

OPERATIVE TREATMENT

Operative management of symptomatic hindfoot arthritis can start with joint debridement, which can have some benefit for pain reduction but usually does not cure the problem. This treatment can be done either via an arthroscopic or mini-open approach. Subtalar arthrodesis, however, is preferred for the treatment of symptomatic subtalar arthritis (**Fig. 8**). The most common indications for subtalar arthrodesis

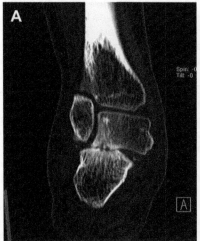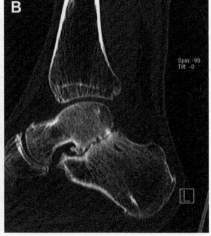

Fig. 7. (*A*) Coronal CT of posttraumatic subtalar arthritis (secondary to a calcaneus fracture). (*B*) Sagittal CT of posttraumatic subtalar arthritis. *Abbreviations:* A, anterior view; L, lateral view.

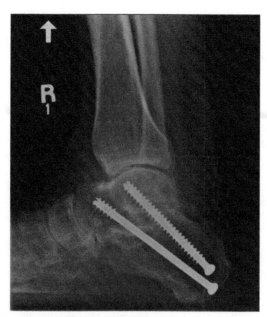

Fig. 8. Lateral radiograph of subtalar arthrodesis.

include subtalar joint arthritis, a residual tarsal coalition, or residual deformity without a fixed forefoot deformity. Mann and colleagues[31] showed that with an isolated subtalar arthrodesis, patients lose half of the normal inversion and eversion of the foot. However, there was minimal progression of arthrosis in the talonavicular and calcaneocuboid joints, and motion in the sagittal plane is maintained.[34] Typically, the heel is usually placed in approximately 5° of valgus, a near physiologic amount. If the heel is put in too much valgus, patients can experience a painful subfibular impingement; if the heel is put in too little valgus or even varus, the transverse tarsal joints are locked and lateral forefoot pressure is increased with gait, causing pain. Multiple studies have shown good fusion rates. Dahm and Kitaoka[42] showed a 93% fusion rates, and Easley and colleagues showed a 96% fusion rate. However, Easley and colleagues excluded smokers, revisions, patients who needed structural grafts, and patients with previous tibiotalar arthrodeses. Mann and Baumgarten[43] evidenced a 93% satisfaction rate at 5 years postoperatively. A bone block can be used as part of the arthrodesis if there is significant loss of calcaneal height secondary to a calcaneal fracture. This bone block increases the talar inclination angle and decreases the anterior tibiotalar impingement.

SUMMARY

Arthritis of the foot and ankle can be a painful and debilitating problem. Initial nonoperative management of the problem can include orthotics, bracing, and corticosteroid injections. Once a problem has progressed to the point when the symptoms are no longer controlled by nonoperative measures, surgical interventions are the typical treatment. These interventions include debridement, osteotomies to realign arthritic joints, and arthrodesis. Other treatments, including interposition arthroplasty and joint replacement, have been tried; but the current data are not supportive of their use.

REFERENCES

1. Administration on Aging. Aging Statistics. 2013. Available at: http://www.aoa.gov/Aging_Statistics/.
2. Furner SE, Hootman JM, Helmick CG, et al. Health-related quality of life of US adults with arthritis: analysis of data from the behavioral risk factor surveillance system, 2003, 2005, and 2007. Arthritis Care Res (Hoboken) 2011;63(6):788–99.
3. Davies-Colley M. Contraction of the metatarsophalangeal joint of the great toe. BMJ 1887;1:728.
4. Cotterill J. Stiffness of the great toe in adolescents. BMJ 1888;1:1158.
5. Coughlin MJ, Mann RA, Saltzman CL. Surgery of the foot and ankle. Philadelphia: Mosby Inc; 2007. p. 867, 869.
6. Gould N, Schneider W, Ashikaga T. Epidemiological survey of foot problems in the continental United States: 1978-1979. Foot Ankle 1980;1(1):8–10.
7. Yee G, Lau J. Current concepts review: hallux rigidus. Foot Ankle 2008;29(6): 637–46.
8. Coughlin MJ, Shurnas PS. Hallux rigidus: demographics, etiology and radiographic assessment. Foot Ankle 2003;24(10):731–43.
9. Deland JT, Williams JR. Surgical management of hallux rigidus. J Am Acad Orthop Surg 2012;20(6):347–58.
10. Coughlin MJ, Shurnas PS. Hallux rigidus: grading and long-term results of operative treatment. J Bone Joint Surg Am 2003;85(11):2072–88.
11. Solan MC, Calder JD, Bendall SP. Manipulation and injection for hallux rigidus: is it worthwhile? J Bone Joint Surg Br 2001;83(5):706–8.
12. Pons M, Alvarez F, Solana J, et al. Sodium hyaluronate in the treatment of hallux rigidus: a single-blind, randomized study. Foot Ankle 2007;22(6):462–70.
13. DuVries HV. Surgery of the foot. St Louis (MO): Mosby Year Book; 1959. p. 392–9.
14. Hattrup SJ, Johnson KA. Subjective results of hallux rigidus following treatment with cheilectomy. Clin Orthop Relat Res 1998;226:182–91.
15. Kennedy JG, Brodsky AR, Gradl G, et al. Outcomes after interposition arthroplasty for treatment of hallux rigidus. Clin Orthop Relat Res 2006;445:210–5.
16. Moberg E. A simple operation for hallux rigidus. Clin Orthop 1979;142:55–6.
17. Easley ME, Hodges Davis W, Anderson RB. Intermediate to long-term follow-up of medial-approach dorsal cheilectomy for hallux rigidus. Foot Ankle 1999;20: 147–52.
18. Keller WL. The surgical treatment of bunions and hallux valgus. New York Med J 1904;80:741–2.
19. Wrighton JD. A ten-year review of Keller's operation. Review of Keller's operation at the Princess Elizabeth Hospital, Exeter. Clin Orthop Relat Res 1974;89: 207–14.
20. Love TR, Whynot AS, Farine I, et al. Keller's arthroplasty: a prospective review. Foot Ankle 1987;8:46–54.
21. O'Doherty DP, Lowrie IG, Magnussen PA, et al. The management of the painful first metatarsophalangeal joint in the older patient: arthrodesis or Keller's arthroplasty. J Bone Joint Surg Br 1990;72:839–42.
22. Hamilton WG, O'Malley MJ, Thompson FM, et al. Capsular interposition arthroplasty for severe hallux rigidus. Foot Ankle 1997;18:68–70.
23. Kennedy JG, Chow FY, Dines J, et al. Outcomes after interposition arthroplasty for treatment of hallux rigidus. Clin Orthop Relat Res 2006;445:210–5.
24. Lau JT, Daniels TR. Outcomes following cheilectomy and interpositional arthroplasty in hallux rigidus foot. Foot Ankle 2001;22:462–70.

25. Barca F. Tendon arthroplasty of the first metatarsophalangeal joint in hallux rigidus: preliminary communication. Foot Ankle Int 1997;18:222–8.
26. Gibson JN, Thomson CE. Arthrodesis or total replacement arthroplasty for hallux rigidus: a randomized controlled trial. Foot Ankle 2005;26(9):680–90.
27. Brodsky JW, Baum BS, Pollo FE, et al. Prospective gait analysis in patients with first metatarsophalangeal joint arthrodesis for hallux rigidus. Foot Ankle 2007; 28(2):162–5.
28. DeFrino PF, Brodsky JW, Pollo FE, et al. First metatarsophalangeal arthrodesis: a clinical, pedobarographic and gait analysis study. Foot Ankle 2002;23(6): 496–502.
29. Hardcastle PH, Reschauer R, Kutscha-Lissberg E, et al. Injuries to the tarsometatarsal joint: incidence, classification and treatment. J Bone Joint Surg Br 1982; 64(3):349–56.
30. Chong M, Sochor M, Ipaktchi K, et al. The interaction of 'occupant factors' on the lower extremity fractures in frontal collision of motor vehicle crashes based on a level I trauma center. J Trauma 2007;62(3):720–9.
31. Mann RA, Prieskorn D, Sobel M. Midtarsal and tarsometatarsal arthrodesis for primary degenerative osteoarthrosis or osteoarthrosis after trauma. J Bone Joint Surg Am 1996;78(9):1376–85.
32. Mukherjee D, Nissen SE, Topol EJ. Risk of cardiovascular events associated with selective COX-2 inhibitors. JAMA 2001;286(8):954–9.
33. Rao S, Baumhauer JF, Becica L, et al. Shoe inserts alter plantar loading and function in patients with midfoot arthritis. J Orthop Sports Phys Ther 2009;39(7): 522–31.
34. Patel A, Rao S, Nawoczenski D, et al. Midfoot arthritis. J Am Acad Orthop Surg 2010;18(7):417–25.
35. Saltzman CL, Johnson KA, Goldstein RH, et al. The patellar tendon-bearing brace as treatment for neurotrophic arthropathy: a dynamic force monitoring study. Foot Ankle 1992;13(1):14–21.
36. Komeda GA, Myerson MS, Biddinger KR. Results of arthrodesis of the tarsometatarsal joints after traumatic injury. J Bone Joint Surg Am 1996;78(11):1665–76.
37. Raikin SM, Schon LC. Arthrodesis of the fourth and fifth tarsometatarsal joints of the midfoot. Foot Ankle 2003;24(8):584–90.
38. Berlet GC, Hodges Davis W, Anderson RB. Tendon arthroplasty for basal fourth and fifth metatarsal arthritis. Foot Ankle 2002;23(5):440–6.
39. Shawen SB, Anderson RB, Cohen BE, et al. Spherical ceramic interpositional arthroplasty for basal fourth and fifth metatarsal arthritis. Foot Ankle 2007;28(8): 896–901.
40. Jung HG, Myerson MS, Schon LC. Spectrum of operative treatments and clinical outcomes for atraumatic osteoarthritis of the tarsometatarsal joints. Foot Ankle 2007;28(4):482–9.
41. Rao SN, Baumhauer J. Midfoot arthritis: nonoperative options and decision making for fusion. Tech Foot Ankle Surg 2008;7:188–95.
42. Dahm DL, Kitaoka HB. Subtalar arthrodesis with internal compression for posttraumatic arthritis. J Bone Joint Surg Br 1998;80(1):134–8.
43. Mann RA, Baumgarten M. Subtalar fusion for isolated subtalar disorders. Clin Orthop Relat Res 1988;(226):260–6.

Ankle Arthritis
Review of Diagnosis and Operative Management

Robert Grunfeld, MD*, Umur Aydogan, MD, Paul Juliano, MD

KEYWORDS

- Ankle • Arthritis • Diagnosis • Operative management

KEY POINTS

- The current standard of care for nonoperative options include the use of nonsteroidal anti-inflammatory drugs, corticosteroid injections, orthotics, and ankle braces. Other modalities, including hyaluronic injections, physical therapy, transcutaneous electrical nerve stimulation units, massage therapy, lack high-quality research studies to delineate the appropriateness and effectiveness of their use.
- The gold standard for operative intervention in end-stage degenerative arthritis remains arthrodesis, but evidence for the equivalence and perhaps even superiority in functional outcomes of total ankle arthroplasty is increasing.
- The next few years will enable us to make more informed decisions, and, with more prospective high-quality studies, the most appropriate patient population for total ankle arthroplasty can be identified.

INTRODUCTION

The ankle joint is the most commonly injured joint in the body and absorbs more force per square centimeter than any other joint. However, the incidence of ankle arthritis is 9 times less common than symptomatic arthritis in the knee and hip.[1] Unlike arthritis in the knee and hip joint, ankle arthritis is most commonly posttraumatic, and primary arthritis remains uncommon. Saltzman and colleagues[2] reported 7.2% of primary ankle arthritis compared with 70% of posttraumatic arthritis, in a sample of 639 patients across a 13-year period. Rheumatoid arthritis was seen in 11.9% of patients.[2]

ANATOMY/PATHOPHYSIOLOGY

Trauma to the ankle joint, including Weber A to C fractures, pilon fractures, and osteochondral injuries to the talus (osteochondritis dissecans [OCD]) as well as lateral ankle

Department of Orthopaedic Surgery, Milton S. Hershey Medical Center, Penn State College of Medicine, Hershey, PA, USA
* Corresponding author.
E-mail address: rgrunfeld@hmc.psu.edu

Med Clin N Am 98 (2014) 267–289
http://dx.doi.org/10.1016/j.mcna.2013.10.005
0025-7125/14/$ – see front matter © 2014 Elsevier Inc. All rights reserved.

ligament sprains/laxity, are the most common contributing factors to the development of ankle arthritis.[1] A rate of 14% of posttraumatic ankle arthritis can be seen with ankle fractures.[3] Weber C fractures can be associated with up to 33% incidence of degenerative changes and the presence of a posterior malleolar fracture, and any associated fracture type increases the risk of arthritis development. Anatomic alignment during reduction decreases the risk for development of arthritis significantly.[3] In an experimental study, sectioning of the deltoid ligament was found to decrease contact area by 15% to 20%, and therefore increase the contact force per area.

Pilon fractures are high-energy intra-articular ankle fractures with a high degree of comminution (**Fig. 1**). These fractures are also associated with the development of ankle arthritis, and damage to the articular cartilage. Open fractures can lead to an additional increased risk of infection and posttraumatic arthritis (**Fig. 2**).[4] Treatment of choice is open reduction internal fixation, but even with an anatomic reduction, this type of injury is associated with a high incidence of degenerative changes.[5] The mean latency time for the development of posttraumatic arthritis was 20.9 years in 1 study.[6] Patients' age (ie, older patients) as well as complications during the treatment of the fracture were related to a shorter latency in the onset of arthritis.[6]

Talar neck fracture can also lead to the development of tibiotalar arthritis, with rates of 47% to 97% described in the literature.[7] Osteochondral injuries to the talus (OCD lesions), whether acquired at the time of an ankle fracture dislocation or of idiopathic origin, predispose patients to the development of ankle arthritis. These lesions are best diagnosed with magnetic resonance imaging (MRI) scans.

It is estimated that symptomatic ankle arthritis is encountered 8 to 9 times less when compared with knee osteoarthritis.[1,8] This estimate translates to 24 times more total knee replacements being performed in the United States compared with total ankle arthroplasty.[1] In a cadaver study using 50 samples, grade 2, 3, or 4 degenerative changes were found in 76% of ankles, compared with 95% of knees.[9]

There are also differences in cartilage properties between different joints. Ankle cartilage is thinner compared with hip or knee cartilage.[10] It ranges from less than 1 mm to approximately 2 mm.[11] The surface contact area for the ankle is also smaller (350 mm²),[12] compared with that of the knee and hip, at 1120 mm² and 1100 mm², respectively.[1] Most of the load is transmitted over the superior portion of the talus, and the ankle joint experiences loads up to 5 times of a person's body weight.[13] In dorsiflexion, the contact area across the talus is largest, and it decreases by 18% in plantarflexion. This finding is associated with an increase in force per unit area.[14]

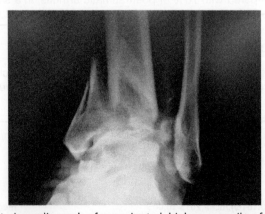

Fig. 1. Anteroposterior radiograph of comminuted, high-energy pilon fracture.

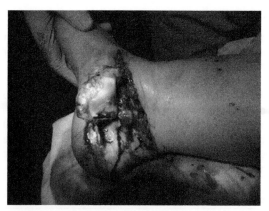

Fig. 2. Open ankle fracture with exposed tibial plafond.

Several unique properties of talar cartilage have been described. The tensile strength of the cartilage seems to undergo fewer age-related changes compared with that of the hip.[15] In addition, the increased congruency of the ankle cartilage seems to make it less likely to undergo changes to cyclical loading.[16] These properties may contribute to the overall lower incidence of primary osteoarthritis of the ankle when compared with that of the hip and knee.

CLINICAL PRESENTATION

Pain and functional limitations are the most common presenting symptoms in patients with ankle arthritis.[17]

Coughlin and colleagues[17] recommend that all patients should be asked the following:

1. Is there a history of trauma?
2. What activities worsen the ankle pain and limit function?

Patient History

The history of trauma, even remote, can be helpful in diagnosing posttraumatic ankle arthritis.[17] The patient should also be asked about recurrent sprains, which they may not immediately recall or associate with a history of trauma. Next, patients need to asked about their medical comorbidities, including rheumatoid arthritis, diabetes, hemophilia, infection, avascular necrosis, and history of previous ankle procedures.[17] Diabetes mellitus, as well as low-bone density, predispose patients to the development of Charcot arthropathy.[18]

Activities

Next, patients should be asked about activities that aggravate their pain and limit their function. Pain that worsens with uphill climbing may be related to the anterior ankle, whereas downhill pain is related to the posterior ankle.[17] Pain on uneven ground is often related to disease in the subtalar joint, whereas pain in the posteromedial joint is often caused by posterior tibial tendon dysfunction (PTTD), and is less related to ankle arthritis.[17] Subfibular or posterolateral ankle pain can be caused by peroneal tendons, or impingement between the calcaneus and talus or fibula. This finding may be seen in the aftermath of calcaneus fractures.[19]

CLINICAL FINDINGS

A complete physical examination includes examination of the patient in both a standing and a sitting position.[17] In addition, gait examination is imperative, as well as examining the patient for hindfoot alignment (ie, varus/valgus heel). Physicians need to take note of any malalignment seen along the lower extremity axis, from hip to knee, and along the tibial shaft. During the gait examination, the examiner needs to note the position of the forefoot during heel strike. When examining patients with flatfoot deformity and PTTD, single and double toe rise needs to be tested. Correction of hindfoot alignment, or lack thereof, indicates late stage PTTD. When the hindfoot remains in valgus during heel rise, a fixed, or stage 3, PTTD can be diagnosed. In these patients, treatment with a fusion procedure is often then indicated.

Sitting Examination

During this part of the examination, the stability of all ankle ligaments is assessed, including anterior talofibular ligament (ATFL) and calcaneofibular ligament (CFL). The ATFL is examined in plantarflexion and the CFL in slight dorsiflexion.[17] The range of motion of the ankle is documented and the Silfverskiöld test is performed, examining for Achilles and gastrocnemius contracture. Improved dorsiflexion with the knee flexed indicates gastrocnemius contracture, whereas limited dorsiflexion with both the knee straight and in a flexed position indicates Achilles contracture. This part of the examination is of particular importance, because it can alter one's operative plan.[17]

Skin and Vascular

A careful skin and vascular examination documenting pulses, capillary refill, and presence of ulcer or calluses is a mandatory component of a complete physical examination. Skin changes may indicate vasculitis, as, for example, in rheumatoid arthritis or complex regional pain syndrome.[17]

DIAGNOSTIC IMAGING

Plain films of the ankle remain the gold standard for initial imaging modality. Standing films of the ankle are preferred, examining anteroposterior, mortise, and lateral views. Radiographs of the foot are also included if surgery in the hindfoot or midfoot is planned as part of the surgical treatment.[17] Saltzman and colleagues[2] also focused on the hindfoot alignment for diagnostic and operative planning purposes. Hindfoot imagining using the Harris view can be easily accomplished in the office setting. Recently, a study[20] reported that the long-axis view of the hindfoot may have better interobserver reliability than the hindfoot alignment view.

Advanced imaging with computed tomography (CT) and MRI scans is appropriate in select settings. CT scans may be used to gain an improved appreciation of posttraumatic changes at the tibiotalar joint, nonunions, and in cases of complex deformity or retained hardware. CT scans are less susceptible to hardware artifacts and motion artifacts compared with MRI. MRI is less frequently used for the diagnosis of ankle arthritis. Its main advantage lies in characterization of the surrounding soft tissues. It can also shed light on the mechanism of injury that led to the development of posttraumatic arthritis.[21] For posttraumatic patients and patients with significant lower extremity deformity, a scanogram can assist in therapeutic and diagnostic decision making.

DIAGNOSTIC TESTING AND PROCEDURES

One of the most important modalities for both diagnostic and therapeutic purposes includes the use of corticosteroid injections into the tibiotalar joint.[17] A positive response to an ankle injection has been found to be predictive of a positive response to surgery.[22] These injections can be completed in the office setting without fluoroscopic guidance (Juliano, personal communication) or can be accomplished under fluoroscopic guidance in the radiology suite. Administration of contrast dye to delineate the joint may be helpful in cases of severe osteoarthritis or in patients with complete varus or valgus deformities.[17] Diagnostic injections with viscosupplementation are less well established and remain more controversial.[23,24]

The location for the injection must be carefully chosen, especially when used for diagnostic purposes.[22] For generalized tibiotalar arthritis, the injection uses the soft tissue depression between the medial malleolus and the medial border of the tibialis anterior. This is a reliable and reproducible location, even in patients with narrowed joint spaces secondary to degenerative disease.[22] A 10-mL syringe with 25-gauge needle (2.54–3.81 cm [1–1.5 in]). One percent lidocaine without epinephrine (3–5 mL) and 1 mL of solumedrol 1 mL celestone can be used. Solumedrol is equivalent to 200 mg hydrocortisone per injection, compared with 150 mg with 1 mL of Celestone.[25]

DIAGNOSTIC DILEMMAS AND DIFFERENTIALS

Ankle arthritis can be classified based on anatomy and underlying cause. In terms of anatomy, arthritis can be global (where the entire tibiotalar joint is affected) or localized (specific portions of the articular surface are affected).[17] The underlying cause of the arthritis can be classified into 3 broad categories: posttraumatic, osteoarthritis, and rheumatoid arthritis; Charcot arthropathy and hemochromatosis; or degenerative changes caused by tumor.[1] The stages of osteoarthritis can be outlined using radiographic parameters:

Stage 0: normal joint, or subchondral sclerosis
Stage 1: presence of osteophytes without joint space narrowing (**Fig. 3**)
Stage 2: joint space narrowing, with or without osteophytes
Stage 3: subtotal or total disappearance or deformation of joint space (**Fig. 4**)

More recently, the Canadian Orthopaedic Foot and Ankle Society (COFAS) classification for end-stage ankle arthritis has been described.[26] The COFAS classification has been shown to have good interobserver reliability ($\kappa = 0.62$) and intraobserver reproducibility ($\kappa = 0.72$). A postoperative classification was developed for the COFAS stages, with even higher interobserver reliability and improved reliability.[27]

PROGNOSIS

Ankle arthritis reduces the number of total steps per day taken by patients, as well high-intensity steps, and is associated with a slower walking speed, when compared with age-matched controls.[28] This situation can have a detrimental impact on patients' activities of daily living (ADLs). The prognosis of ankle arthritis can be self-limiting, but some patients can experience a continued decline in their activity level and an increase in their pain. Besides a decrease in the number of steps taken by patients, studies have also found decreased ankle range of motion and decreased plantar flexion power during gait analysis.[28]

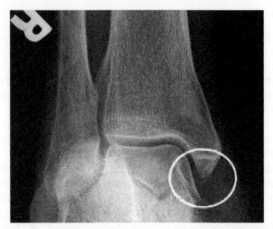

Fig. 3. Anteroposterior view of a right ankle. A medial osteophyte is circled. This is an example of a stage 1 ankle with degenerative changes. Presence of osteophytes without joint space narrowing.

MANAGEMENT GOALS

The goal of management is pain control, improvement of patient's function and ADLs, and a decrease in their level of pain.

PHARMACOLOGIC STRATEGIES
Nonsteroidal Antiinflammatory Drugs

The most common pharmacologic strategy addressing ankle arthritis is nonsteroidal antiinflammatory drugs (NSAIDs). The side effects of NSAIDs require judicious

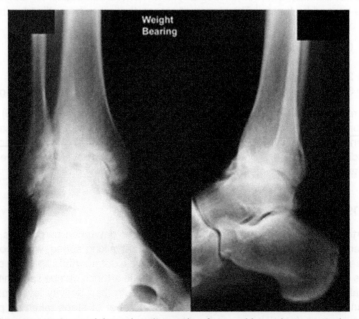

Fig. 4. Anteroposterior and lateral radiograph of an ankle with stage 3 degenerative changes. Subtotal or total disappearance or deformation of joint space.

prescribing and use. These side effects can include gastrointestinal bleeding, stroke, and increased cardiovascular risks.[29] Recent recommendations have focused on the use of topical NSAIDs, particular in high-risk patients for localized osteoarthritis.[29] All patients need to be carefully screened for comorbidities before the initiation of an NSAID regimen.[17,29] Based on our clinical experience, the efficacy of NSAIDs varies and is patient dependent.

Corticosteroid Injections and Viscosupplementation

Tibiotalar joint injections with corticosteroids continue to be 1 final nonsurgical option that patients can be offered in the office setting after failing NSAID therapy and activity modifications. Although corticosteroid injections remain the gold standard, there are an increased number of research articles examining the role of viscosupplementation with hyaluronate in ankle arthritis.[23,24,30] In a more recent study,[31] 3 weekly injections of hyaluronate resulted in pain relief, decreased acetaminophen consumption, and improvement of balance tests. Patients were followed up to 6 months, with improvements in their American Orthopaedic Foot and Ankle Society (AOFAS) scores noted.

   Risks of the injection need to be explained to the patient and all questions answered. These risks include injection site reactions, infections, risk of damage to articular cartilage, and permanent skin depigmentation.[32] Several clinicians have experienced the unpleasant effect of permanent skin discoloration and the patient dissatisfaction that can accompany this.

NONPHARMACOLOGIC STRATEGIES
Self-Management Strategies

Activity modifications can be one of the most effective strategies in early ankle arthritis.[17] By avoiding uneven platforms (ie, subtalar arthritis), uphill climbs (anterior ankle arthritis), and using treadmills or elliptical exercise machines to continue to stay active, patients can achieve some pain control.

Orthotics

Another effective strategy seems to be mechanical unloading of the joint.[17] This strategy can be accomplished via ankle foot orthosis, based on either ankle or calf lacers.[33] Lace-up ankle support can be especially effective in patients who experience instability or mechanical misalignment.[1] Rocker-bottom shoes with the addition of a solid ankle cushioned heel can be worn.[34] Additional strategies include a temporary plaster or fiber-glass cast, or the use of a CAM walker boot. These options can be selected based on both patient preference and financial resources available. Other nonsurgical, nonpharmacologic options include physical therapy modalities, chiropractic care, and acupuncture. There are few peer-reviewed studies or reviews on these modalities.

SURGICAL TECHNIQUE

When patients have failed conservative treatment options, surgical approaches to ankle arthritis can be considered. The most common surgical options include:

1. Arthroscopy
2. Corrective osteotomies
3. Distraction arthroplasty
4. Ankle arthrodesis
5. Total ankle arthroplasty

The goals of surgery are similar to nonsurgical options: pain relief and improve or stabilize function. Based on the stage and location of arthritis (global vs localized), as well as patient demographics, surgical options include arthroscopic debridement, supramalleolar osteotomy, distraction arthroplasty, arthrodesis, and total ankle arthroplasty.[1,17] There are numerous techniques and approaches for tibiotalar arthrodesis, with no clear empiric evidence of 1 technique being superior in terms of outcomes compared with others.

Arthroscopy

Ankle arthroscopy along with debridement has several indications in ankle arthritis. Patients with loose bodies, early degenerative changes, and osteochondral lesions may be suitable candidates for arthroscopy.[17] In addition, impinging osteophytes can often be addressed with ankle arthroscopy. A recent review of the available evidence provides the following list of indications for ankle arthroscopy: ankle impingement, osteochondral lesions, and arthroscopy for ankle arthrodesis.[35] Contraindications include isolated advanced ankle arthritis, excluding the presence of a specific lesion or osteophyte leading to impingement.[35–37]

Supramalleolar Osteotomy

Supramalleolar osteotomies address fracture malunions and malalignment of the lower extremity, which contribute to ankle arthritis.[1] In addition, in posttraumatic arthritis, seen in fractures with partial or complete articular involvement, supramalleolar osteotomies can be of benefit.[1] Varus ankle alignment can be treated with a medial opening-wedge osteotomy or a lateral closing-wedge osteotomy. Patients who had a lower preoperative talar tilt (<7.3°) and neutral or varus heel alignment were more likely to experience outcomes that were associated with improved AOFAS score and radiographic ankle congruence.[38] However, a common cause of failure and recurrence of the deformity lies in the articular involvement. One of the pitfalls can be seen in the posttraumatic varus ankle, with medial plafond involvement. When the articular defect is not addressed with the osteotomy, recurrence of the deformity after an osteotomy may lead to a salvage procedure, such as a fusion or ankle replacement.[39] To address this, Mann and colleagues[39] proposed an intra-articular medial osteotomy (plafond-plasty). In this case series, only 4 of 19 patients required revision to an ankle fusion or a replacement during the follow-up period. A statistically significant deformity correction from an average of 16° varus, to 10° postoperatively, alongside an improvement in AOFAS scores was seen with the plafond-plasty. The plafond-plasty was accompanied with reconstructions of the lateral ligaments.[39]

Distraction Arthroplasty

The use of ankle arthroscopy and debridement, followed by the application of an external fixator with an applied distraction force across the joint, is termed distraction arthroplasty.[1] The original description of the procedure included distraction of the ankle joint by 1 mm per day, for up to a total of 5 mm.[40] Patients were allowed to bear full weight on the fixator, which was converted to a hinged external fixator at 6 weeks. Removal of the hinged fixator occurred at an average of 15 weeks. Results did not show a change in ankle range of motion, but at the 3-year follow-up, a 27% increase in joint space was noted.[41] Most of the data come from a single European physician group and should be interpreted with the limitations inherent to this. Tellisi and colleagues[42] reported that only 2 of 23 patients underwent ankle arthrodesis after distraction arthroplasty, with a follow-up of 30 months after frame removal, and 91% reporting improved pain. In another case series, Paley and colleagues[43] reported that only 1 patient out of 32 required a fusion, and 78% of patients maintained their ankle range of motion at follow-up. However, the most current review of the literature,[44] including a 2012 level of evidence study, indicates that there is no sufficiently high-quality, well-designed research to make a recommendation for or against its use on posttraumatic ankle arthritis. Further research using long-term, high-quality designs is needed to guide our clinical practice.

Arthrodesis

Tibiotalar arthrodesis

Tibiotalar arthrodesis is perhaps one of the most established and well-studied operative treatments of end-stage tibiotalar arthritis. The main indication for fusion of the ankle joint is failed conservative therapy in patients with intractable pain or deformity of the ankle joint.[1,17] Posttraumatic osteoarthritis remains the most common underlying cause.[1,45] Other causes include idiopathic osteoarthritis, avascular necrosis, history of osteomyelitis (not active), failed total ankle arthroplasty,[46,47] postpolio syndrome, congenital deformities,[17] and rheumatoid arthritis.[1] Thomas and Daniels[1] do not recommend arthrodesis as a primary salvage procedure for acute trauma. One of the main advantages of arthrodesis is the reliability of pain relief after successful surgery. In addition, the need for implant or hardware removal is decreased with arthrodesis. Ankle arthrodesis can be accomplished via, open, arthroscopic or with the use of the Ilizarov technique. Regardless of the particular approach used to fuse the ankle, the most important factor in a successful operation is ankle position and soft tissue handling.[17]

Ankle position during arthrodesis The currently accepted position of the ankle is neutral dorsiflexion, 5° of hindfoot valgus and external rotation in 5° to 10°.[1,48] Other researchers have recommended a position of external rotation that mimics the rotation of the contralateral extremity. At heel strike, the midfoot plantarflexes 10° during normal gait.[49] With the ankle fused in a neutral position, this motion is allowed to occur. Fusion in equinus leads to the development of a gait abnormality during heel strike, because the midfoot is unable to dorsiflex. Hefti and colleagues[48] also recommended placing the talus backward in relation to the tibia and fusing it in 5° to 10° of external rotation. This strategy has the theoretic advantage of improved push-off via the natural pronation mechanism.

Soft tissue handling Soft tissue handling is of vital importance when performing arthrodesis. This procedure includes careful retraction, and releasing retractors at every opportunity to decrease insult to the soft tissues, avoiding scar contractures and areas of erythema.[17] Cutaneous nerves need to be protected whenever possible, and planned incision and meticulous dissection techniques are paramount. For the anterior arthrotomy, branches of the superficial peroneal nerve are most at risk, whereas the sural nerve is in danger during a lateral approach and around the lateral malleolus.

Internal versus external fixation Internal fixation remains the first choice during arthrodesis for most patients. Advantages over external fixation include a higher fusion rate and decreased inconvenience for patients.[50] The nonunion rate is cited as 5% for internal fixation, compared with 21% in the external fixation group.[50] Infections were also more common in the external fixator group, at 5 of 28 patients (pin track infections), compared with no superficial or deep infections in the internal fixation group.[50]

Plates versus screws

Several previous studies have shown improved compression with the use of screws compared with plate fixation.[51–55] An additional advantage of screws is decreased soft tissue stripping compared with plates.[1] T-plate fixation for fusions may offer advantages in certain situations.[56] Cadaver biomechanical testing showed that T-plate fixation provided the greatest stiffness compared with screw fixation or fibular strut graft.[56,57] In osteopenic bone, the option of using 2 plates in anterolateral and anteromedial positions may offer improved fixation strength and fusion rates.[58] In 1 cadaver study,[58] bending stiffness was improved by 1.5 to 2 times compared with using a single anterior plate. Commercial systems are available using anterior, lateral, and posterior plating options.

Screw configuration

The use of 2 crossed screws produces increased rigidity compared with parallel screws.[59] One possible screw configuration used at our institution is shown in **Fig. 5**.

Number of screws

Studies have shown that 3 screws can provide increased stiffness compared with 2 screws.[60] The stability of the fusion can further be enhanced with the use of a fibular strut graft.[61] Several techniques for the specific approach and screw configuration have been described. Holt and colleagues[52] described the use of 3 screws along with a fibular osteotomy. Kish and colleagues[62] described a technique using cannulated screw fixation. This technique allows for 3 to 4 screws to be placed, with the aid of guidewires to ensure satisfactory alignment and correction of deformity compression across the fusion site (**Fig. 6**).[63]

External Fixations

The main indication for external fixation is during active infections and in patients with compromised soft tissues.[1] In addition, in severe osteoporosis, in which decreased screw purchase and compression across the fusion site is possible, external fixation may be the preferred modality.[1] This technique allows for immediate weight bearing as tolerated and can be used as a salvage approach.[64]

Internal Versus External Fixation

Internal fixation has several advantages over external fixation, including a higher reported fusion rate and decreased inconvenience for patients.[50] The nonunion rate is cited as 5% for internal fixation, compared with 21% in the external fixation group.[50] Infections were also more common in the external fixator group at 5 of 28 patients (pin track infections), compared with no superficial or deep infections in the internal fixation group.[50]

Gait Analysis in Ankle Arthrodesis

Thomas and Daniels[1] provide a thorough review of the main points with regards to alterations in the gait cycle. Overall, the energy expenditure during walking is increased by 3%.[65]

TOTAL ANKLE ARTHROPLASTY

Four devices are currently approved by the US Food and Drug Administration (FDA) for total ankle arthroplasty: Agility, Salto, Scandinavian Total Ankle Replacements (STAR), and INBONE. The third generation of total ankle arthroplasty is in use. The use of ankle arthroplasty started in the 1970s.[1] It is becoming widespread in North America, but

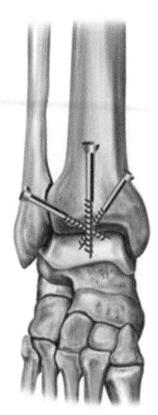

Fig. 5. Tibiotalar arthrodesis. Technique using 3 cannulated, partially threaded screws. After cartilage is denuded and the fusion bed is prepared, alignment corrections are made. Initial fixation is performed using a K-wire, followed by (1) Medial to lateral: medial to lateral direction, aiming from superior to inferior. Guidewire is kept in place under fluoroscopy. Measure with depth gauge. Use a washer for this screw to place screw under compression. Back out guidewire. (2) Anterior to posterior: anterior tibia into posterior talus. (3) Syndesmotic screw: for additional stability, make a lateral stab incision, place lateral fibula to medial talar screw, stabilizing the syndesmosis. This screw is placed percutaneously through the stab incision.

has been popular and well established in Europe. Most ankle replacements used outside the United States are mobile bearing, whereas most used within the United States are fixed bearing.

INDICATIONS

One of the current challenges is controversy in the indications for this procedure and identifying the most appropriate patients who will benefit in the short-term and long-term. Surgical candidates are adult patients who have failed several months of conservative treatment and have end-stage degenerative joint disease of the ankle. The following prerequisites should be fulfilled: (1) adequate vascular flow to the extremity and (2) an adequate soft tissue envelope around the ankle to allow for wound healing and the initiation of physical therapy and ankle range of motion exercises postoperatively.[66–68]

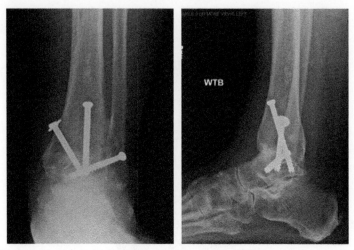

Fig. 6. Tibiotalar arthrodesis. Technique using 3 cannulated, partially threaded screws. Sixteen-week postoperative films obtained in the clinic. A solid fusion mass across the ankle joint is noted, with intact hardware.

CONTRAINDICATIONS TO TOTAL ANKLE ARTHROPLASTY

Contraindications for total ankle arthroplasty include infection, osteonecrosis of the talus, severe malalignment, compromised soft tissue, severe laxity, and neurologic dysfunction.[1] Coetzee and Deorio[69] recommend that a valgus deformity of more than 20° is prohibitive for a total ankle replacement. These investigators also recommend that foot deformities need to be addressed and treated at or before the time of the arthroplasty, because foot deformities can lead to early implant failure. Severe valgus deformities, as seen in end-stage adult acquired flatfoot deformity, can be addressed at the time of total ankle replacement. This is especially the case in patients who had previous fusion procedures in the midfoot or hindfoot (**Fig. 7**).

Types of total ankle replacement (total ankle arthroplasties can be classified along several different parameters)[70]:

I. Fixation: fixation can be cemented or uncemented
II. Number of components: the number of components ranges from 2 to 3; these components can be congruent or incongruent; congruency refers to incongruent (trochlear, bispherical, concave/convex) to congruent (spherical, cylindrical, conical)
III. Constraint: constrained, semiconstrained, or nonconstrained
IV. Component shape: nonanatomic versus anatomic
V. Bearing: fixed or mobile

Agility Ankle

The Agility ankle is a 2-component design system with fixed bearings. This is a semiconstrained device and allows for 60° of motion.[71] This design includes a syndesmotic fusion, with the goal to prevent subsidence of the tibial component.[70] Both the talus and tibia are nonanatomic, with a porous coated talus. Claridge and Sagherian[72] reviewed some of the intermediate-term results of the Agility ankle. Improvements in AOFAS score were seen from 34.9 to 76.4, preoperative to postoperative, respectively. The

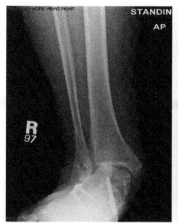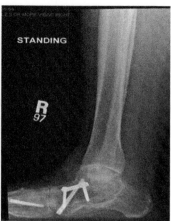

Fig. 7. A pantalar arthritis with previous midfoot fusions and an already fused subtalar joint. There is valgus malalignment and the tibiotalar, subtalar, and midfoot joints are involved. In this case, the subtalar joint and midfoot joints are fused and are stable. This situation enables us to address the valgus deformity as well as the end-stage arthritis at the tibiotalar joint with an ankle arthroplasty, as opposed to a tibiotalocalcaneal fusion.

investigators were concerned regarding the high rate of complications, ranging from superficial to deep infections, iatrogenic fractures, and arterial injury to patients requiring free flap coverage. At a follow-up of 9 years, 11% of patients required revisions (132 arthroplasties in 126 patients were reviewed). Other studies reported survival rates range from 80% to 95% at 5 years and 63% at 10 years.[73,74] The most promising results of 2-component systems include 85% survival at 10 years.[75] The incidence of subtalar arthritis was 19%, and 16% of patients had progressive talonavicular arthritis.[72] In 8% of patients, nonunion of the syndesmosis was seen.[76]

Salto

This is a mobile-bearing system, used in Europe since 1997 (**Fig. 8**). This system includes a conical talus fixed with pegs and a flat tibial component with fin fixation.[70] Survival rate of 65% at 6.8 years was reported in a study including 96 implants in 92 patients. The most common causes for failures resulting in reoperations included bone cysts (11 patients), polyethylene fractures (5 patients), and unexplained pain (3 patients).[77]

STAR

STAR is an uncemented, hydroxyapatite-coated total ankle prosthesis (**Fig. 9**). This system includes a cylindrical talus and a flat tibial component.[78] It was approved by the FDA on May 27, 2009. The 5-year survival of this prosthesis ranges from 70%[66] to 89.5%, with a 10-year survival of 71.1%.[79] The postoperative range of motion was found to be equivalent to the postoperative range of motion.[79] Zhao and colleagues[79] cautioned about the higher rate of loosening that is seen with the STAR prosthesis in their study.

INBONE

This 2-component system was FDA approved in 2005. It includes a titanium-based tibial component with a cobalt-chromium talus. The tibial component includes an

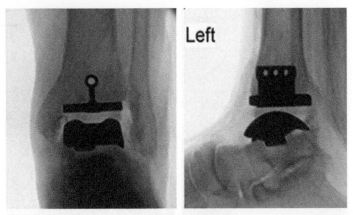

Fig. 8. Total ankle arthroplasty using the Salto implant. This is a mobile-bearing system. The talus has a conical shape and is fixed with pegs. The tibial component is flat and includes a fin for fixation.

intramedullary stem.[80] This design feature requires intramedullary reaming under fluoroscopy and a specialized foot holder for the procedure. A newly designed form of this prosthesis called Prophecy has been introduced into the market. With this implant, the ankle CT of the patient is used to produce patient-specific cutting guides using three-dimensional printing and has the advantages of decreasing the operation time and increasing the accuracy of bone cuts.

TOTAL ANKLE VERSUS ARTHRODESIS

In select groups of patients, total ankle arthroplasty may achieve safe, equivalent results compared with arthrodesis and may even lead to improved functional outcomes compared with fusions.[66,80] Haddad and colleagues[67] examined differences between total ankle arthroplasty and arthrodesis. This examination included 852 patients with

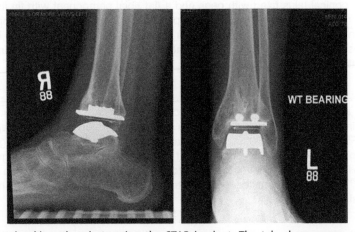

Fig. 9. Total ankle arthroplasty using the STAR implant. The talus has a more cylindrical shape. The tibial component is flat. This is an uncemented prosthesis, coated in hydroxyapatite.

total ankles and 1262 with fusions. A revision rate of 7% in total ankle replacements compared with 9% in fusions was not found to be significant. Salvage procedures were also compared, and 1% of patients with total ankle replacements required a below knee amputation (BKA) compared with 5% in the fusion group.[67] Range of motion may also be improved in ankle replacements compared with arthrodesis.[78] There may also be a smaller rate of degenerative joint changes in adjacent joints with arthroplasty compared with arthrodesis.[81,82]

SURGICAL COMPLICATIONS

In all open foot and ankle procedures, infections, both superficial and deep, remain a concern. Infection rates ranging from less than 2%[55] to 2.5%[51] and up to more than 20% have been described.[83] Delayed wound healing and infection can be addressed and prevented through meticulous soft tissue handling, decreasing retractor force and time, as well as closing of the extensor retinaculum.[1] This strategy can be especially important in total ankle arthroplasty, in which exposed hardware can occur as a result of wound dehiscence.

COMPLICATIONS OF ANKLE ARTHRODESIS

Moeckel and colleagues[50] described the most common complications of arthrodesis as "nonunion, delayed union, stress fracture, infection." Nonunion or pseudoarthrosis may occur with rates ranging from 0% up to 41%.[4,17,53] In several other studies, nonunion rates of less than 10% have been reported.[84,85] Smoking is one of the most recognized factors contributing to nonunion and is associated with a 4 times greater risk of nonunion.[86] Other factors implicated in nonunion are infection, noncompliance with postoperative weight-bearing restrictions, avascular necrosis of the talus, and surgeon technique.[1,86] Frey and colleagues[4] also identified medical comorbidities and history of open fractures as predisposing risk factors for nonunions.

Neurovascular injury and adjacent joint arthritis in the hindfoot and midfoot have also been reported.[1] Radiographic evidence of degenerative changes in the subtalar joint is frequently observed but is commonly clinically asymptomatic.[1] Rates of up to 30% of subtalar osteoarthritis have been observed at 7-year follow-up studies.[87] Although the ipsilateral foot is often involved, the ipsilateral knee seems to be spared from degenerative changes related to the ankle fusion.[82]

COMPLICATIONS OF ARTHROSCOPIC ARTHRODESIS

The most common complication in arthroscopic fusion is painful hardware, resulting in secondary procedures for removal.[17,88] In a study of 42 patients, Crosby and colleagues[89] examined complications of arthroscopic arthrodesis, which included nonunion (7%), iatrogenic fractures (4.8%), pin site infections (9.5%), and painful hardware (9.5%), as well as painful subtalar joints (9.5%), for an overall complication rate of 55%. In a recent meta-analysis of the literature,[90] results of 244 patients were analyzed. A nonunion rate of 8.6% was reported. Of these patients, 66.7% were symptomatic from their nonunion.

COMPLICATIONS OF ANKLE ARTHROPLASTY

The most common complications and reasons for failure of total ankle replacements include aseptic loosening, malalignment, and deep infection (1%).[79,91] These 3 complications accounted for approximately 50% of the failures seen in 1 study review of the literature.[91]

Aseptic loosening and implant failure is multifactorial. Limb and hindfoot deformities can be a contributing factor in many cases.[1] Guidelines have previously been proposed with regards to alignment issues in total ankle arthroplasty.[1] These guidelines include careful examination of preoperative radiographs to identify valgus/varus deformities of the hindfoot. Addressing issues these either before or at the time of the ankle replacement is vital to ensuring longevity of the implant. Obtaining full-length standing films to look for knee and tibia malalignment is also important. Supramalleolar osteotomies for distal tibia deformities greater than 10° have previously been recommended.[92]

Failure of total ankle arthroplasty can have drastic consequences for patients. Deep infection of a prosthesis often necessitates removal of the implant, irrigation and debridement, long-term antibiotics, possible antibiotic spacer placement, and consideration of several salvage options.[1] Compared with ankle arthrodesis, more extensive bone cuts are made during ankle replacements, and revision procedures and salvage options must take this diminished bone stock into account. This situation often leaves fewer options available after failed total ankle arthroplasty, including revision arthroplasty, ankle arthrodesis, and BKA.[93,94] Recent meta-analyses have examined the conversion of failed total ankle arthroplasty to ankle arthrodesis, with Haddad and colleagues[67] reporting a 5.1% conversion rate, and Stengel and colleagues[95], a 6.3% rate.[95]

EVALUATION, ADJUSTMENT, RECURRENCE

Both total ankle arthroplasty and ankle fusion have led to decrease in pain and improvement in patient function. In a recent study, successful surgery was not related to a decrease in patient's body mass index, who were classified as overweight or obese.[96]

For total ankle arthroplasty, anticipated revision surgery, without hardware exchange, is accepted by many foot and ankle surgeons as the reality.[78] These

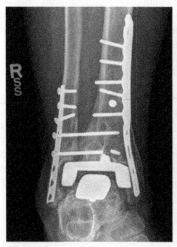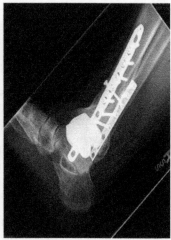

Fig. 10. Mortise radiograph of right ankle of a patient with posttraumatic tibiotalar arthritis, previous open reduction and internal fixation fibula and tibia. Ankle arthroplasty with extensive osteolysis laterally and medially. Scalloping, radiolucent area around the prosthesis is noted.

reoperations may include cyst removal, lateral or medial gutter debridement because of pain or impingement, and polyethylene exchange because of wear.[78] If symptoms persist, infection workup using erythrocyte sedimentation rate and C-reactive protein laboratory markers can be initiated. If these tests are negative, revision total ankle arthroplasty can be considered, taking bone stock and soft tissue envelope into account. Osteolysis and polyethylene wear can affect total ankle arthroplasty (**Fig. 10**). Coughlin and colleagues[17] recommend polyethylene exchange, curettage and bone grafting of the osteolytic lesions, and implant inspection for irregular surface wear, which may necessitate complete implant removal and revision.

For ankle arthrodesis, persistence of symptoms after the 12-month period warrants examination for possible nonunion or infection. If results are negative, advanced imaging with CT scans can elucidate subtle nonunion, which may not be evident on plain

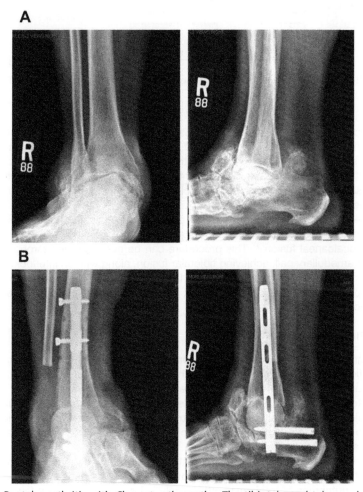

Fig. 11. Pantalar arthritis with Charcot arthropathy. The tibiotalar, subtalar, and midfoot joints are involved. There is also varus malalignment. This deformity can be addressed with a tibiotalocalcaneal fusion. Preoperative (A) and postoperative (B) radiographs are shown.

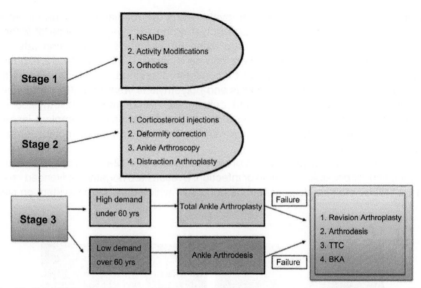

Fig. 12. Flowchart of treatment options at the different stages of ankle arthritis. TTC, tibiotalocalcaneal fusion.

radiographs. Malunion in varus or valgus can be addressed with closing-wedge osteotomies, which has the function of not stretching nerves and providing additional bone for the fusion site.[17] Adjacent joint arthritis in the subtalar joint can be addressed with subtalar arthrodesis, although Coughlin and colleagues[17] caution that the standard 1-screw approach may be insufficient in patients with a preexisting ankle arthrodesis.

If patients have failed previous ankle arthroplasty and failed ankle fusions and advanced degenerative changes in the subtalar joint, a possible salvage procedure is tibiotalocalcaneal fusion.[97] This procedure can be accomplished through a retrograde intramedullary nail, achieving tibiotalar fusion, along with an interlocking screw or blade option for the subtalar joint (**Fig. 11**). Complications have included several reports of periprosthetic fractures in the tibia, proximal to the nail. Intraoperative fracture have also been reported.

DISCUSSION/SUMMARY

The diagnostic and therapeutic options for ankle arthritis are reviewed. **Fig. 12** provides a flowchart of treatment options at the different stages of ankle arthritis.

The current standard of care for nonoperative options include the use of NSAIDs, corticosteroid injections, orthotics, or ankle braces. Other modalities, including hyaluronic injections, physical therapy, transcutaneous electrical nerve stimulation units, massage therapy, lack high-quality research studies to clearly delineate the appropriateness and effectiveness of their use.

The gold standard for operative intervention in end-stage degenerative arthritis remains arthrodesis, but evidence for the equivalence and perhaps even superiority in functional outcomes of total ankle arthroplasty is increasing. The next few years will enable us to make more informed decisions and with more prospective high-quality studies, the most appropriate patient population for total ankle arthroplasty can be identified.

REFERENCES

1. Thomas RH, Daniels TR. Ankle arthritis. J Bone Joint Surg Am 2003;85-A(5): 923–36.
2. Saltzman CL, Salamon ML, Blanchard GM, et al. Epidemiology of ankle arthritis: report of a consecutive series of 639 patients from a tertiary orthopaedic center. Iowa Orthop J 2005;25:44–6.
3. Lindsjo U. Operative treatment of ankle fracture-dislocations. A follow-up study of 306/321 consecutive cases. Clin Orthop Relat Res 1985;(199):28–38.
4. Frey C, Halikus NM, Vu-Rose T, et al. A review of ankle arthrodesis: predisposing factors to nonunion. Foot Ankle Int 1994;15(11):581–4.
5. Marsh JL, Buckwalter J, Gelberman R, et al. Articular fractures: does an anatomic reduction really change the result? J Bone Joint Surg Am 2002; 84(7):1259–71.
6. Horisberger M, Valderrabano V, Hintermann B. Posttraumatic ankle osteoarthritis after ankle-related fractures. J Orthop Trauma 2009;23(1):60–7.
7. Daniels TR, Smith JW. Talar neck fractures. Foot Ankle 1993;14(4):225–34.
8. Huch K, Kuettner KE, Dieppe P. Osteoarthritis in ankle and knee joints. Semin Arthritis Rheum 1997;26(4):667–74.
9. Muehleman C, Bareither D, Huch K, et al. Prevalence of degenerative morphological changes in the joints of the lower extremity. Osteoarthr Cartil 1997;5(1): 23–37.
10. Shepherd DE, Seedhom BB. Thickness of human articular cartilage in joints of the lower limb. Ann Rheum Dis 1999;58(1):27–34.
11. Athanasiou KA, Niederauer GG, Schenck RC Jr. Biomechanical topography of human ankle cartilage. Ann Biomed Eng 1995;23(5):697–704.
12. Cushnaghan J, Dieppe P. Study of 500 patients with limb joint osteoarthritis. I. Analysis by age, sex, and distribution of symptomatic joint sites. Ann Rheum Dis 1991;50(1):8–13.
13. Stauffer RN, Chao EY, Brewster RC. Force and motion analysis of the normal, diseased, and prosthetic ankle joint. Clin Orthop Relat Res 1977;(127):189–96.
14. Calhoun JH, Li F, Ledbetter BR, et al. A comprehensive study of pressure distribution in the ankle joint with inversion and eversion. Foot Ankle Int 1994;15(3): 125–33.
15. Kempson GE. Age-related changes in the tensile properties of human articular cartilage: a comparative study between the femoral head of the hip joint and the talus of the ankle joint. Biochim Biophys Acta 1991;1075(3):223–30.
16. Muehleman C, Berzins A, Koepp H, et al. Bone density of the human talus does not increase with the cartilage degeneration score. Anat Rec 2002;266(2):81–6.
17. Coughlin MJ, Mann RA, Saltzman CL. Surgery of the foot and ankle. 8th edition. Philadelphia: Mosby; 2007.
18. Herbst SA, Jones KB, Saltzman CL. Pattern of diabetic neuropathic arthropathy associated with the peripheral bone mineral density. J Bone Joint Surg Br 2004; 86(3):378–83.
19. Banerjee R, Saltzman C, Anderson RB, et al. Management of calcaneal malunion. J Am Acad Orthop Surg 2011;19(1):27–36.
20. Reilingh ML, Beimers L, Tuijthof GJ, et al. Measuring hindfoot alignment radiographically: the long axial view is more reliable than the hindfoot alignment view. Skeletal Radiol 2010;39(11):1103–8.
21. Kavanagh EC, Zoga AC. MRI of trauma to the foot and ankle. Semin Musculoskelet Radiol 2006;10(4):308–27.

22. Khoury NJ, el-Khoury GY, Saltzman CL, et al. Intraarticular foot and ankle injections to identify source of pain before arthrodesis. AJR Am J Roentgenol 1996;167(3):669–73.
23. Sun SF, Chou YJ, Hsu CW, et al. Efficacy of intra-articular hyaluronic acid in patients with osteoarthritis of the ankle: a prospective study. Osteoarthr Cartil 2006; 14(9):867–74.
24. Mei-Dan O, Kish B, Shabat S, et al. Treatment of osteoarthritis of the ankle by intra-articular injections of hyaluronic acid: a prospective study. J Am Podiatr Med Assoc 2010;100(2):93–100.
25. Tallia AF, Cardone DA. Diagnostic and therapeutic injection of the ankle and foot. Am Fam Physician 2003;68(7):1356–62.
26. Krause FG, Di Silvestro M, Penner MJ, et al. Inter- and intraobserver reliability of the COFAS end-stage ankle arthritis classification system. Foot Ankle Int 2010; 31(2):103–8.
27. Krause FG, Di Silvestro M, Penner MJ, et al. The postoperative COFAS end-stage ankle arthritis classification system: interobserver and intraobserver reliability. Foot Ankle Spec 2012;5(1):31–6.
28. Segal AD, Shofer J, Hahn ME, et al. Functional limitations associated with end-stage ankle arthritis. J Bone Joint Surg Am 2012;94(9):777–83.
29. Roth SH, Anderson S. The NSAID dilemma: managing osteoarthritis in high-risk patients. Phys Sportsmed 2011;39(3):62–74.
30. Witteveen AG, Giannini S, Guido G, et al. A prospective multi-centre, open study of the safety and efficacy of hylan G-F 20 (Synvisc) in patients with symptomatic ankle (talo-crural) osteoarthritis. Foot Ankle Surg 2008;14(3):145–52.
31. Sun SF, Hsu CW, Sun HP, et al. The effect of three weekly intra-articular injections of hyaluronate on pain, function, and balance in patients with unilateral ankle arthritis. J Bone Joint Surg Am 2011;93(18):1720–6.
32. Jones A, Doherty M. Intra-articular corticosteroids are effective in osteoarthritis but there are no clinical predictors of response. Ann Rheum Dis 1996;55(11): 829–32.
33. Saltzman CL, Shurr D, Kamp J, et al. The leather ankle lacer. Iowa Orthop J 1995;15:204–8.
34. Wagner FW Jr. Ankle fusion for degenerative arthritis secondary to the collagen diseases. Foot Ankle 1982;3(1):24–31.
35. Glazebrook MA, Ganapathy V, Bridge MA, et al. Evidence-based indications for ankle arthroscopy. Arthroscopy 2009;25(12):1478–90.
36. Feder KS, Schonholtz GJ. Ankle arthroscopy: review and long-term results. Foot Ankle 1992;13(7):382–5.
37. Amendola A, Petrik J, Webster-Bogaert S. Ankle arthroscopy: outcome in 79 consecutive patients. Arthroscopy 1996;12(5):565–73.
38. Lee WC, Moon JS, Lee K, et al. Indications for supramalleolar osteotomy in patients with ankle osteoarthritis and varus deformity. J Bone Joint Surg Am 2011; 93(13):1243–8.
39. Mann HA, Filippi J, Myerson MS. Intra-articular opening medial tibial wedge osteotomy (plafond-plasty) for the treatment of intra-articular varus ankle arthritis and instability. Foot Ankle Int 2012;33(4):255–61.
40. van Valburg AA, van Roermund PM, Lammens J, et al. Can Ilizarov joint distraction delay the need for an arthrodesis of the ankle? A preliminary report. J Bone Joint Surg Br 1995;77(5):720–5.
41. Marijnissen AC, Van Roermund PM, Van Melkebeek J, et al. Clinical benefit of joint distraction in the treatment of severe osteoarthritis of the ankle: proof of

concept in an open prospective study and in a randomized controlled study. Arthritis Rheum 2002;46(11):2893–902.

42. Tellisi N, Fragomen AT, Kleinman D, et al. Joint preservation of the osteoarthritic ankle using distraction arthroplasty. Foot Ankle Int 2009;30(4):318–25.

43. Paley D, Lamm BM, Purohit RM, et al. Distraction arthroplasty of the ankle–how far can you stretch the indications? Foot Ankle Clin 2008;13(3):471–84, ix.

44. Smith NC, Beaman D, Rozbruch SR, et al. Evidence-based indications for distraction ankle arthroplasty. Foot Ankle Int 2012;33(8):632–6.

45. Scranton PE Jr. An overview of ankle arthrodesis. Clin Orthop Relat Res 1991;(268):96–101.

46. Kitaoka HB, Romness DW. Arthrodesis for failed ankle arthroplasty. J Arthroplasty 1992;7(3):277–84.

47. Carlsson AS, Montgomery F, Besjakov J. Arthrodesis of the ankle secondary to replacement. Foot Ankle Int 1998;19(4):240–5.

48. Hefti FL, Baumann JU, Morscher EW. Ankle joint fusion–determination of optimal position by gait analysis. Arch Orthop Trauma Surg 1980;96(3):187–95.

49. King HA, Watkins TB Jr, Samuelson KM. Analysis of foot position in ankle arthrodesis and its influence on gait. Foot Ankle 1980;1(1):44–9.

50. Moeckel BH, Patterson BM, Inglis AE, et al. Ankle arthrodesis. A comparison of internal and external fixation. Clin Orthop Relat Res 1991;(268):78–83.

51. Chen YJ, Huang TJ, Shih HN, et al. Ankle arthrodesis with cross screw fixation. Good results in 36/40 cases followed 3-7 years. Acta Orthop Scand 1996;67(5):473–8.

52. Holt ES, Hansen ST, Mayo KA, et al. Ankle arthrodesis using internal screw fixation. Clin Orthop Relat Res 1991;(268):21–8.

53. Maurer RC, Cimino WR, Cox CV, et al. Transarticular cross-screw fixation. A technique of ankle arthrodesis. Clin Orthop Relat Res 1991;(268):56–64.

54. Mann RA, Rongstad KM. Arthrodesis of the ankle: a critical analysis. Foot Ankle Int 1998;19(1):3–9.

55. Morgan CD, Henke JA, Bailey RW, et al. Long-term results of tibiotalar arthrodesis. J Bone Joint Surg Am 1985;67(4):546–50.

56. Dohm MP, Benjamin JB, Harrison J, et al. A biomechanical evaluation of three forms of internal fixation used in ankle arthrodesis. Foot Ankle Int 1994;15(6):297–300.

57. Scranton PE Jr, Fu FH, Brown TD. Ankle arthrodesis: a comparative clinical and biomechanical evaluation. Clin Orthop Relat Res 1980;(151):234–43.

58. Kestner CJ, Glisson RR, Nunley JA 2nd. A biomechanical analysis of two anterior ankle arthrodesis systems. Foot Ankle Int 2013;34(7):1006–11.

59. Friedman RL, Glisson RR, Nunley JA 2nd. A biomechanical comparative analysis of two techniques for tibiotalar arthrodesis. Foot Ankle Int 1994;15(6):301–5.

60. Ogilvie-Harris DJ, Fitsialos D, Hedman TP. Arthrodesis of the ankle. A comparison of two versus three screw fixation in a crossed configuration. Clin Orthop Relat Res 1994;(304):195–9.

61. Thordarson DB, Markolf KL, Cracchiolo A 3rd. Arthrodesis of the ankle with cancellous-bone screws and fibular strut graft. Biomechanical analysis. J Bone Joint Surg Am 1990;72(9):1359–63.

62. Kish G, Eberhart R, King T, et al. Ankle arthrodesis placement of cannulated screws. Foot Ankle 1993;14(4):223–4.

63. Natwick JR, Boffeli TJ. A simple technique for cannulated screw fixation. J Foot Ankle Surg 1999;38(4):303–4.

64. Hawkins BJ, Langerman RJ, Anger DM, et al. The Ilizarov technique in ankle fusion: a preliminary report. Bull Hosp Jt Dis 1993;53(4):17–21.
65. Waters RL, Barnes G, Husserl T, et al. Comparable energy expenditure after arthrodesis of the hip and ankle. J Bone Joint Surg Am 1988;70(7):1032–7.
66. Anderson T, Montgomery F, Carlsson A. Uncemented STAR total ankle prostheses. Three to eight-year follow-up of fifty-one consecutive ankles. J Bone Joint Surg Am 2003;85-A(7):1321–9.
67. Haddad SL, Coetzee JC, Estok R, et al. Intermediate and long-term outcomes of total ankle arthroplasty and ankle arthrodesis. A systematic review of the literature. J Bone Joint Surg Am 2007;89(9):1899–905.
68. Saltzman CL, Mann RA, Ahrens JE, et al. Prospective controlled trial of STAR total ankle replacement versus ankle fusion: initial results. Foot Ankle Int 2009; 30(7):579–96.
69. Coetzee JC, Deorio JK. Total ankle replacement systems available in the United States. Instr Course Lect 2010;59:367–74.
70. Hintermann B, Barg A, Knupp M, et al. Conversion of painful ankle arthrodesis to total ankle arthroplasty. J Bone Joint Surg Am 2009;91(4):850–8.
71. Alvine FG. Total ankle arthroplasty: new concepts and approaches. Contemp Orthop 1991;22(4):397–403.
72. Claridge RJ, Sagherian BH. Intermediate term outcome of the agility total ankle arthroplasty. Foot Ankle Int 2009;30(9):824–35.
73. Gougoulias NE, Khanna A, Maffulli N. History and evolution in total ankle arthroplasty. Br Med Bull 2009;89:111–51.
74. Hosman AH, Mason RB, Hobbs T, et al. A New Zealand national joint registry review of 202 total ankle replacements followed for up to 6 years. Acta Orthop 2007;78(5):584–91.
75. Takakura Y, Tanaka Y, Sugimoto K, et al. Ankle arthroplasty. A comparative study of cemented metal and uncemented ceramic prostheses. Clin Orthop Relat Res 1990;(252):209–16.
76. Knecht SI, Estin M, Callaghan JJ, et al. The Agility total ankle arthroplasty. Seven to sixteen-year follow-up. J Bone Joint Surg Am 2004;86(6):1161–71.
77. Bonnin M, Gaudot F, Laurent JR, et al. The Salto total ankle arthroplasty: survivorship and analysis of failures at 7 to 11 years. Clin Orthop Relat Res 2011; 469(1):225–36.
78. Easley ME, Adams SB Jr, Hembree WC, et al. Results of total ankle arthroplasty. J Bone Joint Surg Am 2011;93(15):1455–68.
79. Zhao H, Yang Y, Yu G, et al. A systematic review of outcome and failure rate of uncemented Scandinavian total ankle replacement. Int Orthop 2011;35(12): 1751–8.
80. Cracchiolo A 3rd, Deorio JK. Design features of current total ankle replacements: implants and instrumentation. J Am Acad Orthop Surg 2008;16(9): 530–40.
81. Fuchs S, Sandmann C, Skwara A, et al. Quality of life 20 years after arthrodesis of the ankle. A study of adjacent joints. J Bone Joint Surg Br 2003;85(7):994–8.
82. Coester LM, Saltzman CL, Leupold J, et al. Long-term results following ankle arthrodesis for post-traumatic arthritis. J Bone Joint Surg Am 2001;83(2):219–28.
83. Grunfeld R, Kunselman A, Bustillo J, et al. Wound complications in thyroxine-supplemented patients following foot and ankle surgery. Foot Ankle Int 2011; 32(1):38–46.
84. Sowa DT, Krackow KA. Ankle fusion: a new technique of internal fixation using a compression blade plate. Foot Ankle 1989;9(5):232–40.

85. Monroe MT, Beals TC, Manoli A 2nd. Clinical outcome of arthrodesis of the ankle using rigid internal fixation with cancellous screws. Foot Ankle Int 1999;20(4): 227–31.

86. Cobb TK, Gabrielsen TA, Campbell DC 2nd, et al. Cigarette smoking and nonunion after ankle arthrodesis. Foot Ankle Int 1994;15(2):64–7.

87. Takakura Y, Tanaka Y, Sugimoto K, et al. Long-term results of arthrodesis for osteoarthritis of the ankle. Clin Orthop Relat Res 1999;(361):178–85.

88. Cameron SE, Ullrich P. Arthroscopic arthrodesis of the ankle joint. Arthroscopy 2000;16(1):21–6.

89. Crosby LA, Yee TC, Formanek TS, et al. Complications following arthroscopic ankle arthrodesis. Foot Ankle Int 1996;17(6):340–2.

90. Abicht BP, Roukis TS. Incidence of nonunion after isolated arthroscopic ankle arthrodesis. Arthroscopy 2013;29(5):949–54.

91. Glazebrook MA, Arsenault K, Dunbar M. Evidence-based classification of complications in total ankle arthroplasty. Foot Ankle Int 2009;30(10):945–9.

92. Conti SF, Wong YS. Complications of total ankle replacement. Clin Orthop Relat Res 2001;(391):105–14.

93. Kitaoka HB. Salvage of nonunion following ankle arthrodesis for failed total ankle arthroplasty. Clin Orthop Relat Res 1991;(268):37–43.

94. Stauffer RN. Salvage of painful total ankle arthroplasty. Clin Orthop Relat Res 1982;(170):184–8.

95. Stengel D, Bauwens K, Ekkernkamp A, et al. Efficacy of total ankle replacement with meniscal-bearing devices: a systematic review and meta-analysis. Arch Orthop Trauma Surg 2005;125(2):109–19.

96. Penner MJ, Pakzad H, Younger A, et al. Mean BMI of overweight and obese patients does not decrease after successful ankle reconstruction. J Bone Joint Surg Am 2012;94(9):e57.

97. Kim BS, Knupp M, Zwicky L, et al. Total ankle replacement in association with hindfoot fusion: outcome and complications. J Bone Joint Surg Br 2010; 92(11):1540–7.

Office-Based Management of Adult-Acquired Flatfoot Deformity

Sara Lyn Miniaci-Coxhead, MD*, Adolph Samuel Flemister Jr, MD

KEYWORDS

- Flatfoot • Nonoperative management • Posterior tibial tendon dysfunction
- Medial ankle pain • Hindfoot valgus • Midfoot abduction

KEY POINTS

- Adult-acquired flatfoot deformity is a common problem, caused by dysfunction of the posterior tibial tendon.
- Early in the disease process, patients present with medial-sided pain and swelling, which eventually progresses to lateral-sided pain as the deformity worsens.
- Nonoperative treatment includes nonsteroidal anti-inflammatory drugs, weight loss, and various forms of bracing and immobilization for symptom control.
- If nonoperative management fails or the deformity worsens, patients may be candidates for surgical intervention.

INTRODUCTION

Adult-acquired flatfoot deformity (AAFD) is defined as a loss of the medial longitudinal arch secondary to failure of the posterior tibial tendon (PTT) and posteromedial soft tissue structures.[1] AAFD was initially known as PTT dysfunction (PTTD), because the condition was thought to be solely caused by failure of the PTT. However, over time, it was recognized that dysfunction and attenuation of the surrounding ligaments also occur, leading to a progressive deformity of the foot.[2]

PTT synovitis was initially described in 1955 by Fowler.[3] He is credited with reporting the first series of 7 patients, in which a tenosynovectomy provided pain relief for patients with tenosynovitis. In 1953, Key reported the first case of a partial PTT rupture. He treated this with debridement and noted that the patient was left with 15% disability of that foot.[1,3] Various theories have been described regarding the origin of PTTD, but the most likely cause is repetitive microtrauma to the tendon, which leads to an inflammatory response and then finally tendon disruption.

Department of Orthopaedics, University of Rochester, 601 Elmwood Avenue, Rochester, NY 14642, USA
* Corresponding author.
E-mail address: Sara_Miniaci@URMC.Rochester.edu

Med Clin N Am 98 (2014) 291–299
http://dx.doi.org/10.1016/j.mcna.2013.10.006
0025-7125/14/$ – see front matter

FOOT ANATOMY

The bony anatomy of the hindfoot consists of the subtalar joint, the talonavicular joint, and the calcaneocuboid joint. The talonavicular and calcaneocuboid joints together are known as the *transverse tarsal joints*.[1]

The posterior tibialis muscle originates from the posterior aspect of the tibia and interosseous membrane. It runs immediately posterior to the medial malleolus and divides into multiple slips, inserting on the navicular tuberosity, the plantar surfaces of the second through fourth metatarsals, and the sustentaculum tali, cuboid, and cuneiforms.[1,3,4] The PTT functions to invert and plantarflex the foot. It is also the primary stabilizer of the medial longitudinal arch and hindfoot, and is responsible for locking the midtarsal joints to assist in effective gait patterns.[5]

The spring ligament, also known as the *calcaneonavicular ligament*, is crucial in supporting the medial arch, and therefore its failure contributes to the development of AAFD. The ligament runs from the anterior portion of the sustentaculum tali to the plantar medial aspect of the navicular.[1] It is thought to have 2 components: a superomedial band and an inferior band. Together, these act as a cradle for the plantar medial aspect of the talar head. As the spring ligament becomes attenuated, or ruptures, the talus can migrate in a plantar and medial fashion, leading to subluxation of the talonavicular joint.[1,2]

The deltoid ligament is the primary medial stabilizer of the tibiotalar joint. It has multiple components, the most important being the distal portion that will blend with the spring ligament and talonavicular joint capsule. This aspect of the ligament is subject to repetitive stress during midstance.[1] As the foot deformity progresses, increased strain is placed on the deltoid, leading eventually to deltoid incompetence and a valgus deformity of the tibiotalar joint.[3]

BIOMECHANICS AND PATHOPHYSIOLOGY OF PTTD

The gait cycle is divided into the stance and swing phases. The stance phase consists of the heel strike, midstance, heel rise, and toe off. The posterior tibialis muscle is considered a stance phase muscle, and is therefore intimately involved in positioning the foot appropriately for a biomechanically sound gait pattern.

During heel strike, the posterior tibialis will eccentrically contract to slow the eversion of the subtalar joint, which will unlock the transverse tarsal joint complex, allowing collapse of the foot. As the foot progresses to the midstance and heel rise phase, the posterior tibialis will contract, causing inversion of the subtalar joint. The action of inversion of the subtalar joint locks the transverse tarsal joints, creating a rigid midfoot. This rigid midfoot creates a lever, allowing the contraction of the gastrocnemius-soleus complex to propel the foot and body forward.[1,3,5]

Multiple forces are involved in the development of PTTD. As the PTT becomes deficient, a valgus deformity of the hindfoot is noted, which is caused by the excessive eversion forces created by an unopposed pull of the peroneus brevis. During the stance phase, the lack of posterior tibialis contraction and eversion of the hindfoot cause the transverse tarsal joints to remain unlocked. This unlocked position prevents formation of the rigid lever arm, which accelerates the degeneration of the spring ligament.[3]

As AAFD progresses, the talus will become plantarflexed, the calcaneus will internally rotate and evert, and the navicular and cuboid will evert. These changes lead to the pathognomonic hindfoot valgus deformity (**Fig. 1**A) and forefoot abduction (see **Fig. 1**B).[3]

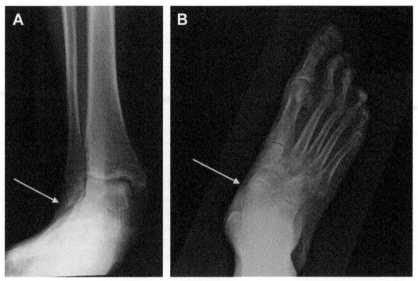

Fig. 1. (*A*) Anteroposterior radiograph of the ankle demonstrating hindfoot valgus and subfibular impingement (*arrow*). (*B*) Anteroposterior radiograph of the foot showing forefoot abduction and uncoverage of the talonavicular joint (*arrow*).

STAGING OF AAFD

In 1989, Johnson and Strom[6] described 3 stages of PTTD. Later, in 1996, Myerson[7] added a fourth stage (**Table 1**). The staging system is based on the amount of deformity of the foot.[1] Stage I is characterized by tenosynovitis of the posterior tibial tendon,

	Definition	Physical Examination	Treatment
		Table 1 **Stages of AAFD**	
	Definition	**Physical Examination**	**Treatment**
Stage I	Tenosynovitis of the PTT Little to no foot deformity	Medial swelling and tenderness Usually able to perform single-leg raise	Bracing, NSAIDs Surgery only indicated in patients refractory to nonoperative management
Stage II	Flexible deformity with collapse at talonavicular joint Elongation and degeneration of PTT	Medial swelling and tenderness Unable to perform single-leg raise	Bracing, NSAIDs Surgery if nonoperative management fails
Stage III	Rigid deformity	Lateral pain greater than medial pain Pain at rest Unable to perform single-leg raise	Nonoperative management for symptom control Surgery usually indicated
Stage IV	Valgus deformity of the talus	Lateral pain secondary to subfibular impingement and arthritis	Usually require surgery

Abbreviation: NSAIDs, nonsteroidal anti-inflammatory drugs.

without any significant deformity. Stage II is defined by a passively correctable deformity. Stage II is further categorized into IIa and IIb, wherein IIa has less than 30% uncoverage of the talonavicular joint, and stage IIb has more than 30% uncoverage. Stage III is a fixed deformity of the foot in valgus and abduction. Finally, stage IV is characterized by concomitant valgus deformity of the ankle joint. The foot deformity can either be flexible (stage IVa) or fixed (stage IVb) (**Fig. 2**).

PATIENT HISTORY AND PHYSICAL EXAMINATION
History

The diagnosis of AAFD is based mostly on history and physical examination. The presenting symptoms can vary according to the stage of the patients' disease. Patients rarely note a traumatic event that precedes the pain, and often an insidious onset of discomfort occurs. Early in the disease process, patients complain of pain and swelling on the medial aspect of the ankle. However, as the tendon fails, the medial pain often dissipates.[2] As the subtalar joint moves into increased valgus, patients begin to complain of lateral pain from subfibular impingement. Standing and walking may aggravate the symptoms, and some will note difficulty with gait, taking longer strides with an inability to push off or raise the heel.[1]

Physical Examination

The physical examination should begin with inspection of the patient in bare feet, noting the alignment of the feet. A cardinal sign of AAFD is the "too many toes

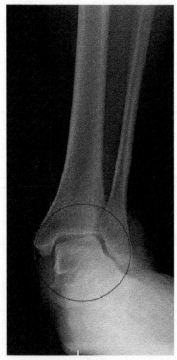

Fig. 2. Anteroposterior radiograph of the ankle demonstrating stage IV AAFD with tibiotalar tilt (*red circle*).

sign." When examining the standing patient from behind, the forefoot abduction will allow the examiner to see more of the lesser toes of that foot (**Fig. 3**).

On palpation, tenderness may be experienced on the medial aspect of the ankle, especially along the course of the posterior tibial tendon. Swelling on the medial side is most often present. Tenderness may also be present laterally in the subfibular region or at the sinus tarsi, depending on the extent of the disease. The passive and active range of motion of the ankle, subtalar, and transverse tarsal joints should be assessed. The strength of the PTT should be assessed with the foot in slight plantar flexion and applying an inversion stress to the first metatarsal. Placing the foot in plantar flexion removes the inversion strength of the anterior tibialis muscle, which must compensate for the incompetent PTT. Often, patients will not be able to invert across the midline. An important evaluation of the integrity of PTT is a single-leg heel raise, which should be performed with the patient standing, and using the wall or table for balance only. The patient is then asked to rise onto the toes one foot at a time, without bending their knee or leaning forward. If the patient is unable to do this, the posterior tibialis tendon is dysfunctional. Finally, a Silfverskiöld test can be performed to evaluate for gastrocnemius-soleus complex contracture. To perform this test, one assesses the patients passive dorsiflexion with the knee flexed and extended. It is important to keep the hindfoot in the neutral position to accurately perform this test. If the dorsiflexion improved when the patient flexes their knee, then the contracture involves the gastrocnemius. If the dorsiflexion remains the same in both knee flexion and extension, the tightness involves the Achilles tendon.

Adult flatfoot caused by PTT insufficiency must be differentiated from flatfoot resulting from other causes, namely congenital flatfoot, tarsal coalition, arthritis, posttraumatic or iatrogenic deformity, Charcot foot, and neuromuscular disorders.[8]

Imaging

Although the diagnosis of PTTD is mostly based on physical examination, radiographic evaluation is also important. Initial films should include weight-bearing views of the foot and ankle. The films must be weight-bearing, because non–weight-bearing films do not give accurate information of the alignment of the foot.[1] Multiple angles can be assessed on the radiographs to determine the presence of a flatfoot deformity.

On the anteroposterior projections of the foot, the talonavicular coverage angle is measured. This angle is between the perpendicular lines to the joint articular margins

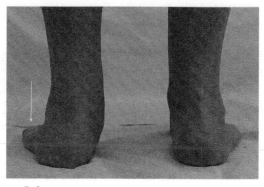

Fig. 3. "Too many toes" sign.

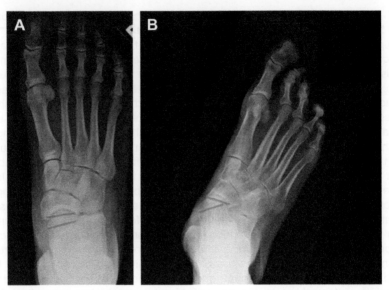

Fig. 4. (A) Normal talonavicular coverage angle (*blue lines*). (B) Increased talonavicular coverage angle as seen in AAFD (*blue lines*).

of the talus and navicular (**Fig. 4**A). If this angle measures greater than 7°, subluxation of the talonavicular joint is present (see **Fig. 4**B).

On the lateral projection of the foot, the talocalcaneal angle, talometatarsal (Meary's) angle, and the cuneiform height should be assessed. The talocalcaneal angle is the angle between the long axis of the talus and the calcaneus, with a normal angle less than 12°. As the flatfoot deformity increases, the talocalcaneal angle increases. The Meary's angle is between the long axis of the talus, and the long axis of the first metatarsal (**Fig. 5**A). This angle ranges between −4° and +4°, with the angle increasing in a flatfoot deformity (see **Fig. 5**B).[3]

Advanced imaging, such as magnetic resonance imaging (MRI), computed tomography (CT) scan, and ultrasound can all be used for further evaluation, although not routinely required. MRI, which is best for assessment of the soft tissues, can be used to evaluate the PTT, spring ligament, deltoid ligament, and muscle. In the acute phase, the PTT may be attenuated, or may be surrounded by fluid, indicating inflammation. A CT scan is best used to evaluate the bony anatomy, and is helpful in evaluating for tarsal coalitions and the presence of arthritis. Finally, ultrasound is a cost-effective and accurate way of evaluating the soft tissues, especially the degenerated PTT.[1,3]

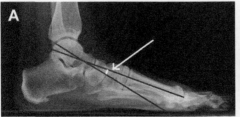
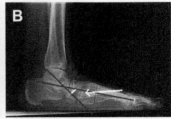

Fig. 5. (A) Normal Meary's (talometatarsal) angle (*arrow*). (B) Increased Meary's angle (*arrow*).

Management

The management of AAFD can be separated into stages. Typically, nonoperative treatment is reserved for stages I and II AAFD, and most clinicians will advocate for a trial of nonoperative management before pursuing surgical intervention for symptom management. The goals of nonoperative management are to decrease patient symptoms and prevent disease progression. Typically, a combination of nonsteroidal anti-inflammatory drugs, weight loss, activity modification, orthotics or bracing, and physical therapy are considered mainstays of initial management.

For stage I deformities, immobilization in a cam walker or ankle stirrup brace for 4 to 6 weeks can help manage symptoms initially.[1] Patients with more severe symptoms may require a short-leg walking cast. After immobilization, patients should be encouraged to use an orthosis. Because patients with stage I AAFD have mild or no deformity, an over-the-counter orthosis with arch support is usually sufficient.

For stage II deformities, a trial of immobilization similar to that used for stage I deformities is helpful for reducing the initial inflammatory response. At this stage, with a more significant deformity, a custom orthosis with medial posting or, in some cases, an over-the-counter arch support is recommended. Patients for whom orthotic management fails may be candidates for more rigid bracing, such as an Arizona ankle-foot orthoses (AFO) (**Fig. 6**).

Stage III AAFD involves a rigid deformity, which cannot be corrected with the use of braces or orthotics. However, these patients may benefit from management with an accommodative AFO designed merely to control residual hindfoot motion.

Nonoperative management of stage IV deformities is similar to that for stage III deformities; however, because stage IV deformities also significantly compromise the tibiotalar joint, surgery should be considered for many of these patients.

The most important aspect of nonoperative treatment is close follow-up to ensure that no progression of the deformity has occurred. If the deformity continues to progress despite intervention, referral to a foot and ankle surgeon is warranted.

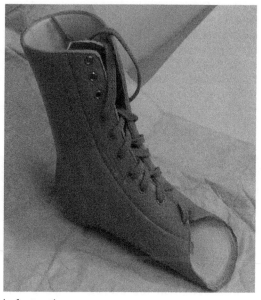

Fig. 6. Arizona ankle-foot orthoses.

To date, limited studies have evaluated the effectiveness of orthoses and bracing on slowing the progression of the deformity. In 2008, a study by Lin and colleagues[9] examined the natural history of the efficacy of nonoperative treatment in patients with stage II disease. They treated patients with an initial period of 6 weeks in a short-leg weight-bearing cast, then transitioned them to a double upright ankle foot orthosis. They found a 69.7% success rate (brace-free and no surgery) at a mean follow-up of 8.6 years. They found the average length of brace wear was 14.2 months, with a mode of 6.0 months. Overall, bracing seems to be somewhat successful in controlling symptoms in patients with stage II disease.

Other studies have focused on the role of physical therapy in the management of AAFD. In 2006, Alvarez and colleagues[10] evaluated patients with stage I or II AAFD with an intact PTT in a rehabilitation program involving orthotics use. They found that most of the patients were globally weak in the long muscles that cross the foot and ankle, and that this weakness improved with a structured rehabilitation program. They reported a success rate of 83%. In 2012, Bek and colleagues[11] published a comparison of patients enrolled in a center-based rehabilitation program versus those undergoing a home-based program. They found that both groups had an increase in strength and range of motion and a decrease in pain. The center-based group had a greater improvement in PTT strength, but both groups were otherwise equal in terms of strength at their final visit.

Finally, Kulig and colleagues,[12] compared a concentric strengthening program with an eccentric strengthening program for stages I and II AAFD. In their series, all patients used orthotics, and their control group was orthotic use only. They used the Foot Functional Index (FFI), a self-reported outcome measure, as their primary outcome. They noted improvement in the FFI across all groups, but the eccentric strengthening group had the most improvement, whereas orthotic use alone had the least.

OPERATIVE TREATMENT

Surgery should be considered for patients with significant pain and disability despite conservative management. Surgery should also be considered in patients with rapidly progressive deformities or those progressing to stage IV.

Surgical intervention involves substitution of the diseased PTT with transfer of another local tendon, usually the flexor digitorum longus. In addition, the bony arch of the foot must be reconstructed.[1] This reconstruction often involves calcaneal osteotomies, fusions, and bone grafting procedures (**Fig. 7**). Typical recovery involves 6 to 8 weeks of no weight-bearing and 3 months of casting, with total recovery occurring after 8 to 12 months. Therefore, it is important to carefully advise patients before surgical intervention.

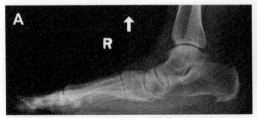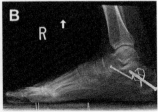

Fig. 7. (A) Preoperative lateral radiograph of the right foot of a patient with AAFD. (B) Postoperative lateral radiograph of the right foot demonstrating of a flatfoot correction, with multiple osteotomies. R, right.

SUMMARY

AAFD is a disabling condition that requires prompt diagnosis and treatment. Initial nonoperative management is reasonable for patients with stages I and II disease, and for some patients with stage III disease. Patients with stage IV disease should be considered for surgical intervention.

REFERENCES

1. Pinney SJ, Lin SS. Current concept review: acquired adult flatfoot deformity. Foot Ankle Int 2006;27:66–75.
2. Deland JT. Adult-acquired flatfoot deformity. J Am Acad Orthop Surg 2008;16: 399–406.
3. Haddad SL, Mann RA. Flatfoot deformity in adults. In: Coughlin MJ, Mann RA, Saltzman CL, editors. Surgery of the foot and ankle. 8th edition. Philadelphia: Mosby Elsevier; 2007. p. 1007–85.
4. Hoppenfeld SP. Surgical exposures in orthopaedics: the anatomic approach. Philadelphia: Lipponcott, Williams, and Wilkins; 2009.
5. Bek N. Home-based general versus center-based selective rehabilitation in patients with posterior tibial tendon dysfunction. Acta Orthop Traumatol Turc 2012;46:286–92.
6. Johnson KA, Strom DE. Tibialis Posterior tendon dysfunction. Clin Orthop Relat Res 1989;239:196–206.
7. Myerson MS. Adult acquired flatfoot deformity: Treatment of dysfunction of the posterior tibial tendon. J Bone Joint Surg Am 1996;78:780–92.
8. Lee MS, Vanore JV, Thomas JL, et al. Diagnosis and treatment of adult flatfoot. J Foot Ankle Surg 2005;44:78–113.
9. Lin JL, Balbas J, Richardson EG. Results of non-surgical treatment of stage II posterior tibial tendon dysfunction: a 7- to 10-year follow-up. Foot Ankle Int 2008;29:781–6.
10. Alvarez RG, Marini A, Schmitt C, et al. Stage I and II posterior tibial tendon dysfunction treated by a structured nonoperative management protocol: an orthosis and exercise program. Foot Ankle Int 2006;27:2–8.
11. Bek N, Simsek IE, Erel S, et al. Home-based general versus center-based selective rehabilitation in patients with posterior tibial tendon dysfunction. Acta Orthop Tramatol Turc 2012;46:286–92.
12. Kulig K, Reischl SF, Pomrantz AB, et al. Nonsurgical management of posterior tibial tendon dysfunction with orthoses and resistive exercise: a randomized controlled trial. Phys Ther 2009;89:26–37.

The Cavus Foot

Andrew J. Rosenbaum, MD*, Jordan Lisella, MD, Nilay Patel, BS,
Nani Phillips, MPH

KEYWORDS

- Cavus foot • Cavovarus foot • Charcot-Marie-Tooth disease • "Peek-a-boo" sign
- Coleman block testing • Meary's angle • Triple arthrodesis

KEY POINTS

- Cavus foot deformity is most often caused by muscle imbalance, with the tibialis posterior and peroneus longus overpowering the peroneus brevis and tibialis anterior, respectively.
- Adult cavus foot deformity has 4 primary causes: neuromuscular, traumatic, and idiopathic processes, and the presence of a residual clubfoot.
- Approximately two-thirds of adults with symptomatic cavus foot have an underlying neurologic abnormality, such as Charcot-Marie-Tooth disease.
- The peek-a-boo sign, a term credited to Beals and Manoli, is a physical examination finding suggesting the presence of a subtle cavus deformity.
- The Coleman block test is an integral part of the physical examination and helps clinicians determine whether the deformity is forefoot- or hindfoot-driven.
- Regardless of the origin, conservative interventions are always attempted first and include accommodative footwear, orthoses, and home stretching programs.
- Surgery is performed when conservative measures fail, with a goal of restoring muscle balance and foot alignment via tendon transfers, corrective osteotomies, and in the most severe cases, arthrodesis.

INTRODUCTION

The cavus, or high-arched, foot was first described in American literature in 1885 by Shaffer.[1] It is now thought to be present in an estimated one-fifth to one-quarter of the population and can present in either childhood or adulthood.[1] Although a multitude of conditions are associated with the cavus foot, it is most frequently considered a manifestation of a neuromuscular process.[2] The other causes include traumatic, congenital, and idiopathic processes.

The cavus foot is one of a wide variety of foot shapes. Although the orthopedic foot and ankle surgeon is often the one to treat the symptomatic cavus foot, general practitioners, family physicians, neurologists, and rheumatologists will all encounter patients with symptomatic high-arched feet. This article provides practitioners with the

Division of Orthopaedic Surgery, Albany Medical Center, Albany, NY 12208, USA
* Corresponding author.
E-mail address: Andrewjrosenbaum@gmail.com

Med Clin N Am 98 (2014) 301–312
http://dx.doi.org/10.1016/j.mcna.2013.10.008
0025-7125/14/$ – see front matter © 2014 Elsevier Inc. All rights reserved.

necessary knowledge to evaluate, diagnose, and treat patients presenting with a cavus foot deformity through an in-depth review of foot and ankle anatomy and biomechanics as they relate to high-arched feet; the associated conditions and underlying origins of cavus deformity; the essential components of the history and physical examination; imaging adjuncts; and treatment modalities.

ANATOMY AND BIOMECHANICS

The proper function of the bones and joints of the foot requires balance between the extrinsic (leg) and intrinsic (foot) muscles of the lower extremity. With muscle imbalance, deformity progressively occurs. Several important muscle pairings balance each other. At the level of the ankle and hindfoot, the tibialis anterior dorsiflexes the first ray, whereas the peroneus longus plantar flexes it; the posterior tibial muscle inverts the hindfoot, whereas the peroneus brevis everts it; and the triceps surae plantarflexes the foot, whereas the tibialis anterior and extensor hallucis longus all work to dorsiflex it.[3] At the level of the forefoot, antagonistic muscle pairings include the intrinsic and extrinsic flexors and extensors of the toes, keeping them straight at the metatarsophalangeal and interphalangeal joints.

During the normal gait cycle, the arch of the foot changes shape. At heel strike, medial rotation of the forefoot and inversion of the heel occurs. In midstance, the subtalar joint assumes a valgus position, unlocking the midtarsal joints and enabling the foot to act as a shock absorber. At the end of the stance phase, there is metatarsophalangeal dorsiflexion and locking of the midtarsal joints, helping the elevated arch to become a rigid lever. The posterior leg muscles ultimately facilitate push-off and provide energy for forward propulsion.

Both forefoot- and hindfoot-driven causes of a cavus foot exist. Forefoot-driven cavus foot is associated with plantarflexion of the first ray. As the foot reaches midstance, this plantarflexion causes the first metatarsal head to contact the ground, in turn stopping the progression of the hindfoot into eversion. This function leads to continued hindfoot varus and an inability of the hindfoot to act as a shock absorber during the remainder of the stance phase of gait. In hindfoot-driven cavus, the abnormality is a primary varus alignment of the hindfoot. Regardless of the cause of the cavus (forefoot or hindfoot), the opposite structure will become a secondary contributor to the cavus deformity over time.

ORIGINS

Adult cavus foot deformity has 4 primary causes: neuromuscular, traumatic, and idiopathic processes, and the presence of a residual clubfoot. The neuromuscular causes include the hereditary motor and sensory neuropathies (HMSNs), cerebral palsy, after effects of stroke, and spinal cord lesions (amyotrophic lateral sclerosis, poliomyelitis, Huntington chorea, Friedreich ataxia). The HMSNs, such as Charcot-Marie-Tooth (CMT) disease, are usually motor, and not progressive or congenital.[4] Approximately two-thirds of adults with symptomatic cavus foot have an underlying neurologic abnormality.[5,6] Muscle imbalance is typically evident in this setting, and traditionally involves relatively strong peroneus longus and tibialis posterior muscles in conjunction with weak tibialis anterior and peroneus brevis muscles. This combination results in a hindfoot varus and forefoot valgus position. Peripheral neuropathy may also cause weakness of the intrinsic muscles, which become overpowered by the long flexors and extensor tendons, causing flexion at the interphalangeal joints and hyperextension at the metatarsophalangeal joints. When this occurs, the thinner, more proximal skin of the plantar foot is brought under the weight-bearing metatarsal head, which can lead to ulceration. Secondary equinus deformity may also develop at the ankle, which can further complicate treatment of the cavus foot. These patients may present with a high-stepping drop-foot gait with hyperextension of the knee.

Foot deformity in patients with cerebral palsy, stroke, or closed-head injury depends on the specific area of motor cortex involved, because this dictates the weakness and spasticity observed. Cavovarus foot deformity is observed in approximately 34% of patients with cerebral palsy. After stroke, equinus and equinovarus deformities frequently occur.[7]

Traumatic causes of cavus foot deformity include compartment syndrome, crush injuries, severe scarring after burns, talar neck fracture malunion, and peroneal nerve injury.[8] In the setting of compartment syndrome of the leg's deep posterior compartment, muscle contractures of the tibialis posterior and flexor digitorum longus may pull the foot into an equinus and cavovarus position.[9] With malunion of the talar neck, a fixed varus position of the subtalar, talonavicular, and calcaneocuboid joints can arise.[10] Peroneal nerve injury can occur after knee dislocation, leading to an equino-cavovarus deformity similar to that seen with compartment syndrome.

Uncorrected or partially treated clubfoot can also lead to the persistence of an equi-nocavovarus foot position.[11] However, in some cases of cavus foot, no underlying cause is found; these instances are termed *idiopathic cavus foot*. The subtle cavus foot is one example of an idiopathic process, because it presents as a foot with a higher arch than normal but is not associated with any specific underlying condition. However, the subtle cavus deformity may be associated with ankle instability, varus ankle arthrosis, peroneal tendon disorders, lateral foot overload with stress fractures, meta-tarsalgia and claw toe deformity, ankle impingement syndromes, plantar fasciitis, lateral knee strain, iliotibial band syndrome, and medial knee arthrosis.

HISTORY AND PHYSICAL EXAMINATION

A careful and thorough history is crucial in evaluating patients with a high-arched foot, because often they have seen other physicians for the same symptoms. Typical complaints include frequent ankle sprains, ankle pain, lateral foot and ankle pain, arch pain, forefoot pain, and, occasionally, knee pain. Patients may also describe difficulty with ambulation, ill-fitting shoes, pain over bony prominences, and painful callosities (**Fig. 1**).

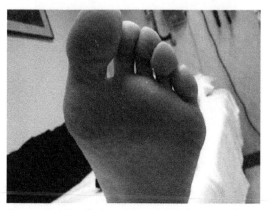

Fig. 1. Heavy callusing under the first metatarsal head, suggesting a cavus foot. (*From* Roberts MM, Greisberg J. Examination of the foot and ankle. In: DiGiovanni CW, Greisberg J, editors. Core knowledge in orthopedics: foot and ankle. Philadelphia: Elsevier; 2007. p. 10–5.)

In patients with residual clubfoot, overload of the cuboid region is often seen secondary to the varus hindfoot and forefoot malalignment. In runners, the cavus foot position leads to increased loading of the metatarsal heads and calcaneus.[12] In the setting of CMT disease, patients may experience increased stress on the lateral border of the foot, the first metatarsal head, or the lateral metatarsal heads. The family history is important when neuromuscular origins are being considered, and clinicians must search for a history of similar diseases between relatives.

The physical examination should involve assessment with the patient sitting, standing, and walking. While seated, the shape and symmetry of the foot and toes should be evaluated; clawing may be present (extension at metatarsophalangeal and flexion at interphalangeal joints) (**Fig. 2**). The skin and soft tissues should be evaluated for

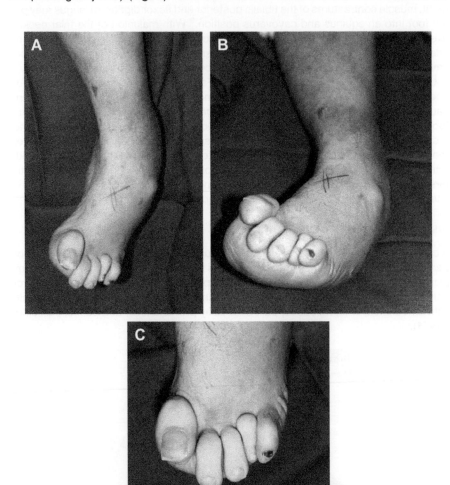

Fig. 2. The left foot of a patient with severe cavovarus deformity. (*A*) The ankle and hindfoot varus. (*B*) Severe clawing. (*C*) The toe deformity has led to injury of the fifth toenail from improper shoe fit. (*From* Greisberg J, Hofstaetter SG, Trnka HJ. Neuromuscular foot deformity. In: DiGiovanni CW, Greisberg J, editors. Core knowledge in orthopedics: foot and ankle. Philadelphia: Elsevier; 2007. p. 67–76.)

lesions and callosities, because longstanding deformity can adversely affect tissue quality. With hindfoot varus, pressure is focused on the lateral border of the foot. This condition can cause pain and callusing, and occasionally fifth metatarsal stress fractures.

A full motor examination should be performed, documenting the strength of each muscle group against active resistance in both legs. Strength can be graded with the Medical Research Council scale or with hand-held dynamometry, which has been found to be an objective instrument for determining muscle strength in the setting of CMT disease.[13] A full sensory and vascular examination must also be performed, and the flexibility of the hindfoot, ankle, and toes is important to assess.

Many conditions begin with a flexible deformity that progressively becomes more rigid over time. When assessing the subtalar joint, any limitations in motion may suggest a coalition or arthrosis. Conversely, when supple subtalar motion is observed in the setting of a cavus foot, a forefoot-driven deformity is most likely present. Gait must be observed, with a foot drop occasionally visible during the swing phase.

The standing evaluation is the most important component of the physical examination. The patient should be facing the practitioner, with the feet parallel and at least 6 inches apart. When a cavus alignment is present, the medial aspect of the heel will be visible when facing forward, suggesting a subtle cavus deformity. This finding was termed the *peek-a-boo* sign by Beals and Manoli.[14] Once varus hindfoot alignment is observed with the patient facing the clinician, evaluation from behind is needed to avoid a false positive peek-a-boo heel sign. This event can occur in patients with large heel pads or in those with severe metatarsus adducts, who externally rotate their lower extremities through the hips to stand facing straight ahead.[15] With the patient facing away from the practitioner, hindfoot alignment should be further assessed. In the normal foot, the heel rests in slight (approximately 5°) valgus, just lateral to the long axis of the tibia. In the presence of a cavus foot, the heel is medially displaced and in varus.

After cavus alignment has been identified, the 1-inch Coleman block test must be performed, because this will help differentiate between forefoot- and hindfoot-driven cavus.[16] While observing the patient from behind, a 1-inch block is placed under the heel and lateral forefoot. The first 2 toes should fall off the medial edge of the block. If the hindfoot corrects to a normal valgus alignment, a forefoot-driven cavus is present and the hindfoot varus is flexible (**Fig. 3**). When little or no correction is observed, the hindfoot is stiff and in varus (**Fig. 4**).

The presence of a gastrocnemius contracture should be noted, because its presence contributes to the forefoot-driven cavus through increasing the relative strength of the peroneus longus compared with the anterior tibialis (**Fig. 5**). Contracture of the gastrocnemius can be evaluated by keeping the hindfoot in a neutral position and dorsiflexing the ankle with the knee extended.[9]

DIAGNOSTIC ADJUNCTS

Imaging should include weight-bearing views of the foot and ankle. The anteroposterior radiograph of the ankles and feet should be taken together on the same plate.[17] The lateral radiograph should include the lower one-third of the leg and foot on one plate. A calcaneal axial view should also be obtained. In the lateral view of a normal foot, the base of the fifth metatarsal and inferior aspect of the medial cuneiform should be near the same level. When the fifth metatarsal base is closer to the floor, the foot is

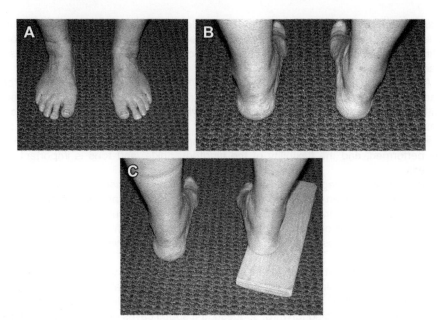

Fig. 3. (*A*) Unilateral cavus foot on the left (patient's right foot). Note the appearance of the medial heel on the left, whereas on the opposite side the medial heel is not visible. (*B*) Right varus heel alignment on the same patient, viewed from behind. (*C*) Correction of heel alignment on Coleman block testing in the same patient. (*From* Chilvers M, Manoli A. The non-neuromuscular cavus foot. In: DiGiovanni CW, Greisberg J, editors. Core knowledge in orthopedics: foot and ankle. Philadelphia: Elsevier; 2007. p. 58–66.)

in cavus (**Fig. 6**). The Meary lateral talometatarsal angle should also be assessed and is measured along the long axis of the talus and first metatarsal. This angle is normally 0°. However, in a cavus foot, the first metatarsal is plantarflexed, which increases the Meary's angle. A Meary's angle of 5° to 10° correlates with a subtle cavus foot, whereas angles greater than 20° are consistent with severe cavus

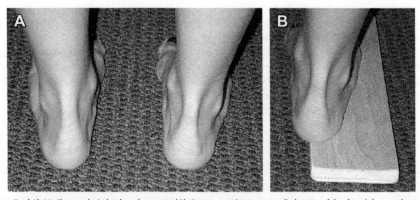

Fig. 4. (*A*) Unilateral right heel varus. (*B*) Same patient on a Coleman block with no change in heel position, indicating hindfoot-driven cavus. (*From* Chilvers M, Manoli A. The non-neuromuscular cavus foot. In: DiGiovanni CW, Greisberg J, editors. Core knowledge in orthopedics: foot and ankle. Philadelphia: Elsevier; 2007. p. 58–66.)

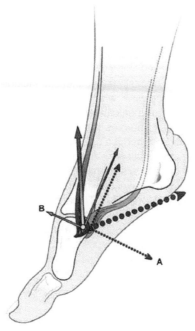

Fig. 5. Peroneus longus contribution to cavus foot alignment is potentiated by equinus ankle position. With the foot in equinus, the relative strength of the peroneus longus (*A*) is greater than the tibialis anterior (*B*), leading to first ray plantar flexion. (*From* Chilvers M, Manoli A. The non-neuromuscular cavus foot. In: DiGiovanni CW, Greisberg J, editors. Core knowledge in orthopedics: foot and ankle. Philadelphia: Elsevier; 2007. p. 58–66.)

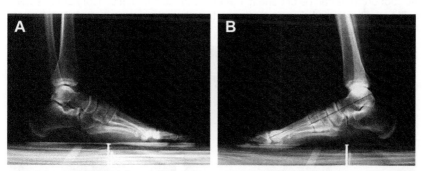

Fig. 6. (*A*) Standing lateral foot-ankle radiograph of a cavus foot. Note the relative height of the medial cuneiform compared with the fifth metatarsal, and the flexion of the long axis of the first metatarsal compared with the long axis of the talus (Meary's angle). (*B*) Standing lateral foot-ankle radiograph of a normal foot. Note that the level of the medial cuneiform is closer to the level of the fifth metatarsal. The long axis of the talus is parallel with the long axis of the first metatarsal. (*From* Chilvers M, Manoli A. The non-neuromuscular cavus foot. In: DiGiovanni CW, Greisberg J, editors. Core knowledge in orthopedics: foot and ankle. Philadelphia: Elsevier; 2007. p. 58–66.)

deformity.[18] Calcaneal pitch is also evaluated on the lateral radiograph, with pitch greater than 30° associated with hindfoot cavus.

A normal anteroposterior radiograph shows a divergent talus and calcaneus, with a talocalcaneal angle of 20° to 40°. When the angle is less and the talus and calcaneus are more parallel, the foot is in cavus (**Fig. 7**). With longstanding cavus feet, the anteroposterior radiograph of the ankle may show the talus to be in varus within the mortise. Other views that are occasionally beneficial include oblique radiographs of the foot and the modified Cobey view, which may provide a more accurate representation of hindfoot alignment than a calcaneal axial view.[19]

Other imaging and diagnostic studies may also be required. A computed tomographic (CT) scan should be obtained if a rigid deformity is present with no correction on Coleman block testing. It can also be used for preoperative planning.[20] Coronal plane reconstructions are of particular benefit for evaluating the axis of the subtalar joint. Sagittal reconstructions effectively delineate Meary's angle and assess the tibiotalar weight-bearing surfaces. However, CT scans provide only a simulated weight-bearing view.[21] Magnetic resonance imaging is infrequently used and is most useful for delineating peroneal tendon abnormalities. If a stress fracture is suspected, nuclear scintigraphy may be of benefit. Electromyography with nerve conduction velocities is used to evaluate patients with a suspected neuromuscular cavus foot to better define the neuromuscular lesion.

CONSERVATIVE TREATMENT

Conservative measures are the first-line treatment for both neuromuscular and non-neuromuscular cavus foot deformity, with a goal of preventing progression of deformity. In the setting of a neuromuscular cavus foot, the underlying disease must be controlled and muscle spasticity treated. Common medications used for this include baclofen, diazepam, and dantrolene. Botulinum toxin blocks may also be helpful. Gastrocnemius stretching programs should also be implemented to prevent the development of contractures. Extradepth shoes are also an effective conservative modality and will help accommodate the high-arched foot. If claw toes are also present, a tall toe box will also be useful. When a weak or unstable ankle is also present, a custom ankle-foot orthosis can be of benefit. Patients with concurrent sensory deficits will also benefit from Plastizote linings in the brace to reduce the recurrence of ulcer formation.

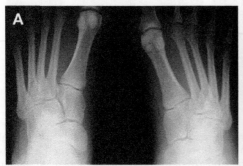 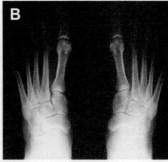

Fig. 7. (*A*) Standing anteroposterior radiograph of a cavus foot. Note the parallelism of the talus and calcaneus. (*B*) Standing anteroposterior radiograph of a normal foot. Note the divergence of the talus and calcaneus. (*From* Chilvers M, Manoli A. The non-neuromuscular cavus foot. In: DiGiovanni CW, Greisberg J, editors. Core knowledge in orthopedics: foot and ankle. Philadelphia: Elsevier; 2007. p. 58–66.)

In the presence of a non-neuromuscular forefoot-driven and supple cavus deformity, a cavus foot orthosis should be tried first (**Fig. 8**). This orthosis has a laterally based forefoot wedge with a recessed area for the first metatarsal head. This design allows for continued first metatarsal plantarflexion and subsequent hindfoot eversion. In a randomized study by Burns and colleagues,[22] patients with custom foot orthoses had a 74% improvement in foot pain, whereas those with simple sham insoles only had a 43% improvement in the setting of cavus deformity. The study attributed the pain relief provided by the custom orthotic devices to the redistribution of pressure from the forefoot and hindfoot to the midfoot. A gastrocnemius stretching program should also be initiated early on, because a tight gastrocnemius potentiates forefoot-driven cavus.

SURGERY FOR THE CAVUS FOOT

Surgery is indicated when conservative measures fail. Cavus deformity can be associated with other problems, such as stress fractures, ankle instability, and peroneal tendon tears. These issues should be addressed first, followed by realignment procedures.

The flexible cavus deformity, which is seen after stroke or head injury, has no bony deformity. Instead, it is solely a function of muscle imbalance and soft tissue contracture. As such, surgery focuses on correcting muscle imbalance. The posterior tibial tendon can be transferred to the dorsum of the foot to augment a weak tibialis anterior, and the peroneus longus can be transferred to the peroneus brevis, helping to restore eversion while also eliminating the strong pull of the longus on the first ray. In stroke patients, transfer of the flexor digitorum longus and flexor hallucis longus tendons anteriorly has been described as an effective intervention.[23]

Mild and subtle cavus deformity presents with a varus hindfoot that stresses the lateral structures of the foot and ankle. Surgical intervention may include all or some of the tendon transfers just described, in addition to osseous realignment procedures. These procedures are dependent on whether the deformity is forefoot- or hindfoot-driven. When a forefoot-driven deformity is present, a first metatarsal dorsiflexion osteotomy can be performed and will usually also correct the secondary hindfoot varus (**Fig. 9**). With hindfoot-driven deformity, a lateralizing calcaneal osteotomy is used to bring the heel out of varus and recreate hindfoot valgus (**Fig. 10**). A first metatarsal dorsiflexion osteotomy may be performed at the same time, particularly if the patient has a symptomatic plantarflexed first ray. When a very stiff cavus foot is

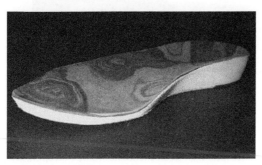

Fig. 8. Cavus foot orthotic. (*From* Chilvers M, Manoli A. The non-neuromuscular cavus foot. In: DiGiovanni CW, Greisberg J, editors. Core knowledge in orthopedics: foot and ankle. Philadelphia: Elsevier; 2007. p. 58–66.)

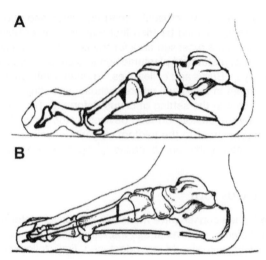

Fig. 9. Illustration of the first metatarsal dorsiflexion osteotomy. (*A*) A dorsally based wedge of bone is removed, approximately 1 cm distal to metatarsocuneiform joint. (*B*) Postoperative illustration depicting a dorsiflexed first metatarsal. (*From* Coughlin MJ, Mann RA. Surgery of the foot and ankle. 7th edition. St Louis (MO): Mosby; 1999. p. 525.)

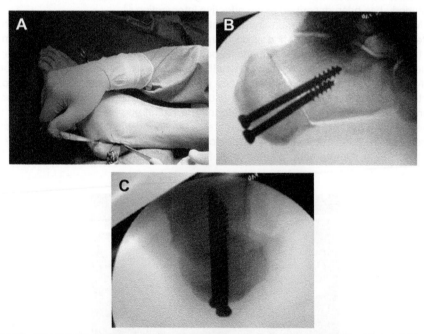

Fig. 10. (*A*) Intraoperative lateralizing calcaneal osteotomy. Postoperative (*B*) and lateral (*C*) radiographs showing the lateralization of the calcaneus and internal fixation. (*From* Chilvers M, Manoli A. The non-neuromuscular cavus foot. In: DiGiovanni CW, Greisberg J, editors. Core knowledge in orthopedics: foot and ankle. Philadelphia: Elsevier; 2007. p. 58–66.)

present, the calcaneal osteotomy can be performed concurrently with a partial medial plantar fasciectomy to ensure sufficient lateralization of the heel.

The fixed cavus deformity is the most severe and can require a triple hindfoot arthrodesis to restore a plantigrade foot. This procedure involves fusion of the subtalar, talonavicular, and calcaneocuboid joints. It is most frequently seen with neuromuscular disease; non-neuromuscular cavus deformity rarely requires arthrodesis. Concomitant deformity (eg, gastrocnemius contracture, claw toes) must also be addressed at the time of surgery for a cavus foot.

SUMMARY

A cavus deformity describes a foot with a higher than normal arch. It is one of several types of foot shapes, including low-, neutral-, and high-arched feet. The orthopedic surgeon is commonly called on to evaluate and treat patients with cavus foot deformity. However, primary care practitioners will also encounter these patients. Cavus foot deformity can be caused by neuromuscular (eg, CMT disease) and non-neuromuscular processes (eg, trauma, idiopathic).

A comprehensive history and physical examination is integral to determining the presence of any underlying abnormality or disease process associated with the foot deformity. Vital components of the examination include evaluation for a peek-a-boo sign, and whether the deformity corrects with Coleman block testing. Weight-bearing anteroposterior and lateral views of the foot and ankle are important imaging studies to obtain and can help to better delineate the severity of the deformity.

Regardless of the underlying cause of a cavus deformity, initial treatment is always conservative. Accommodative footwear, orthoses, and home stretching programs are commonly tried. When these measures fail, operative intervention may be indicated. Both soft tissue and osseous procedures may be performed, all with the goal of restoring normal foot alignment. The specific procedures performed are influenced by the severity of the deformity and whether it is forefoot- or hindfoot-driven. In the most severe cases, triple arthrodesis is indicated.

REFERENCES

1. Ledoux WR, Shofer JB, Ahroni JH, et al. Biomechanical differences among pes cavus, neutrally aligned and pes planus feet in subjects with diabetes. Foot Ankle Int 2003;24:845–50.
2. Sachithanandam V, Joseph B. The influence of footwear on the prevalence of flat foot. A survey of 1846 skeletally mature persons. J Bone Joint Surg Br 1995;77(2): 254–7.
3. Tynan MC, Klenerman L, Helliwell TR, et al. Investigation of muscle imbalance in the leg in symptomatic forefoot pes cavus: a multidisciplinary study. Foot Ankle 1992;13:489–501.
4. Holmes JR, Hansen ST Jr. Foot and ankle manifestations of Charcot-Marie-Tooth disease. Foot Ankle 1993;14:476–86.
5. Lutter LD. Cavus foot in runners. Foot Ankle 1981;1:225–8.
6. Alexander IJ, Johnson KA. Assessment and management of pes cavus in Charcot-Marie-Tooth disease. Clin Orthop 1989;246:273–81.
7. Tenuta J, Shelton YA, Miller F. Long-term follow-up of triple arthrodesis in patients with cerebral palsy. J Pediatr Orthop 1993;13:713–6.
8. Fulkerson E, Razi A, Tejwani N. Review: acute compartment syndrome of the foot. Foot Ankle Int 2003;24:180–7.

9. Younger AS, Hansen ST. Adult cavovarus foot. J Am Acad Orthop Surg 2005;13: 302–15.

10. Sangeorzan BJ, Wagner UA, Harrington RM, et al. Contact characteristics of the subtalar joint: the effect of talar neck misalignment. J Orthop Res 1992;10: 544–51.

11. Haasbeck JF, Wright JG. A comparison of the long-term results of posterior and comprehensive release in the treatment of clubfoot. J Pediatr Orthop 1997;17: 29–35.

12. Sneyers CJ, Lysens R, Feys H, et al. Influence of malalignment of feet on the plantar pressure pattern in running. Foot Ankle Int 1995;16:624–32.

13. Burns J, Redmond A, Ouvrier R. Quantification of muscle strength and imbalance in neurogenic pes cavus, compared to health controls, using hand-held dynamometry. Foot Ankle Int 2005;26:540–4.

14. Beals TC, Manoli A. The "peek-a-boo" heel sign in the evaluation of hindfoot varus. Foot 1996;6:205–6.

15. Manoli A II, Graham B. The subtle cavus foot, "the underpronator," a review. Foot Ankle Int 2005;26:256–63.

16. Coleman SS, Chesnut WJ. A simple test for hindfoot flexibility in the cavovarus foot. Clin Orthop 1977;123:60–2.

17. Chadha H, Pomeroy GC, Manoli A. Radiologic signs of unilateral pes planus. Foot Ankle Int 1997;18:603–4.

18. Paulos L, Coleman SS, Samuelson KM. Pes cavovarus. Review of a surgical approach using selective soft-tissue procedures. J Bone Joint Surg Am 1980; 62:942–53.

19. Saltzman CL, El-Khoury GY. The hindfoot alignment view. Foot Ankle Int 1995;16: 624–32.

20. Liggio FJ, Kruse R. Split tibialis posterior tendon transfer with concomitant distal tibial derotational osteotomy in children with cerebral palsy. J Pediatr Orthop 2001;21:95–101.

21. Van Bergeyk AB, Younger A, Carson B. CT analysis of hindfoot alignment in chronic lateral ankle instability. Foot Ankle Int 2002;23:37–42.

22. Burns J, Crosbie J, Ouvrier R, et al. Effective orthotic therapy for the painful cavus foot: a randomized controlled trial. J Am Podiatr Med Assoc 2006;96:205–11.

23. Yamamoto H, Okumura S, Morita S, et al. Surgical correction of foot deformities after stroke. Clin Orthop 1992;282:213–8.

Ankle Sprains and Instability

Cory M. Czajka, MD[a,*], Elaine Tran, BS[b], Andrew N. Cai, MSc[b],
John A. DiPreta, MD[c]

KEYWORDS

- Sprain • Syndesmosis • Inversion • Eversion • Ottawa ankle rules • PRICEMMMS

KEY POINTS

- Ankle injuries generally are among the most common injuries presenting to primary care providers and emergency departments and may cause considerable time lost to injury and long-term disability.
- Inversion injuries about the ankle involve about 25% of all injuries of the musculoskeletal system and 50% of all sports-related injuries.
- Medial-sided ankle sprains occur much less frequently than those on the lateral side. This is partly because of inversion injuries occurring more frequently but also because of the strength of the medial-sided ligaments.
- High ankle sprains, also known as syndesmotic injuries, involve the distal tibiofibular syndesmosis. They occur less frequently in the general population, but do occur commonly in collision sports.
- Providers should apply the Ottawa ankle rules when radiography is indicated and refer fractures and more severe injuries to orthopedic surgery as needed.

INTRODUCTION

Ankle injuries generally are among the most common injuries presenting to primary care providers and emergency departments.[1] Of these, patients with ankle sprains (stretching of, partial rupture of, or complete rupture of at least one ligament about the ankle) comprise a large percentage of these injuries. Worldwide, approximately 1 ankle sprain occurs per 10,000 person-days, and approximately 2 million acute ankle sprains occur each year in the United States alone.[2] It has been estimated that the annual aggregate health care cost of acute ankle sprains and their treatment approaches $2 billion.[3] Ankle sprains can result in considerable time lost to injury, as well as long-term disability in up to 60% of patients.[4,5] Among younger, more athletic populations ankle sprains account for up to 30% of injuries overall.[2]

[a] Division of Orthopaedic Surgery, Albany Medical College, 43 New Scotland Avenue, Albany, NY 12208, USA; [b] Albany Medical College, 43 New Scotland Avenue, Albany, NY 12208, USA; [c] Division of Orthopaedic Surgery, Capital Region Orthopaedic Group, Albany Medical College, 1367 Washington Avenue, Suite 200, Albany, NY 12206, USA
* Corresponding author. 98 Middlesex Court, Slingerlands, NY 12159.
E-mail address: coryczajka@gmail.com

Med Clin N Am 98 (2014) 313–329
http://dx.doi.org/10.1016/j.mcna.2013.11.003
0025-7125/14/$ – see front matter © 2014 Elsevier Inc. All rights reserved.
medical.theclinics.com

By definition, ankle sprains constitute an injury to 1 or more ligaments about the ankle joint. These, like all ligaments in the human body, serve to provide mechanical stability, proprioceptive information, and directed motion for the joint. Recurrent ankle sprains potentially lead to functional instability of the joint, loss of normal ankle kinematics, and proprioception. Repeated ligamentous injuries may result in chronic instability, degenerative bony changes, and chronic pain.[6]

EPIDEMIOLOGY OF ANKLE SPRAINS

As stated, acute ankle sprain is one of the most common reasons for primary care office and emergency department visits in the United States.

- An overall incidence of 2.15 per 1000 person-years.[2]
- Teenagers and young adults have the highest rates, with a peak incidence of 7.2 per 1000 person-years for those 15 to 19 years of age.[2]
- Nearly one-half of all ankle sprains occur during athletic activity, basketball being the most common sporting activity.[7]
- The greatest risk factor for ankle sprain is a previous ankle sprain.[8]

REVIEW OF RELEVANT ANATOMY ABOUT THE ANKLE JOINT

The ankle joint, or talocrural region, is the region where the leg and foot articulate. The ankle joint is a complex of 3 articulations:

- The talocrural joint is the articulation between the tibia and fibula (proximally) and the talus (distally).
- The distal tibiofibular joint (tibiofibular syndesmosis) is the articulation between the medial side of the distal end of the fibula and the lateral side of the distal end of the tibia.
- The subtalar (talocalcaneal) joint is the articulation between the inferior aspect of the talus and the superior aspect of the calcaneus.

The boney arch formed by the tibial plafond, along with the medial malleolus (the distal-most aspect of the tibia) and lateral malleolus (the distal-most aspect of the fibula), is referred to as the ankle "mortise" (**Figs. 1** and **2**).

SIGNS AND SYMPTOMS OF ACUTE ANKLE SPRAINS

Common signs and symptoms of acute ankle sprains include the following:

- Pain
- Difficulty with weight bearing
- Tenderness
- Significant swelling
- Ecchymosis[8]

Assessment of an acute ankle sprain begins with a complete history and physical. A focused history should begin with the mechanism of injury, as this will direct the rest of the examination toward the ligaments at greatest risk for injury and the extent of injury.

Patients who suffer complete ligament rupture often describe immediate swelling, inability to continue physical activity, and inability to bear weight. Those suffering ligament sprains often describe delayed onset of swelling and the ability to bear weight while continuing physical activity.[9]

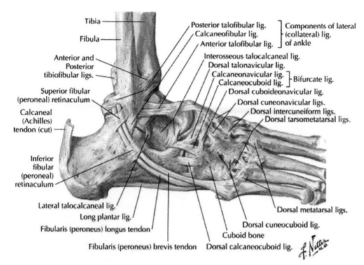

Fig. 1. Basic anatomy of the lateral aspect of the ankle. (Netter illustration from www. netterimages.com. © Elsevier Inc. All rights reserved.)

MECHANISMS OF INJURY

The nature and extent of ankle sprains depends on the mechanism of injury. Athletes most commonly suffer lateral ankle sprains.[10] Inversion injuries about the ankle involve approximately 25% of all injuries of the musculoskeletal system and 50% of

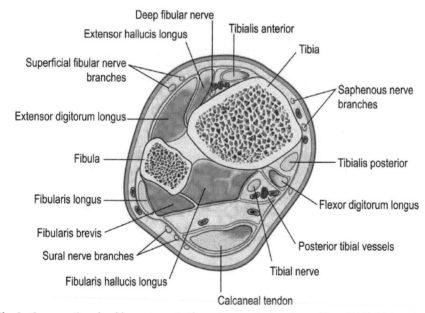

Fig. 2. Cross-sectional ankle anatomy in the anteroposterior plane. (*From* Wells M. Local and regional anesthesia in the emergency department made easy. 1st edition. Edinburgh, New York: Churchill Livingstone; 2010; with permission.)

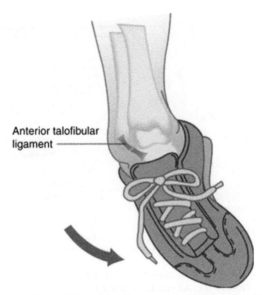

Anterior talofibular
ligament

Fig. 3. Inversion injury of the right ankle. (*From* DeLee JC, Drez D, Miller MD. DeLee and Drez's orthopedic sports medicine. Philadelphia: Saunders; 2010; with permission.)

all sports-related injuries.[9] These injuries most commonly result from excessive inversion of the foot combined with external rotation of the leg (**Fig. 3**).

Inversion injuries typically cause damage to the lateral ligamentous complex of the ankle, which consists of the anterior talofibular ligament (ATFL), the calcaneofibular ligament (CFL), and the posterior talofibular ligament (PTFL).

The ligaments affected depend on the force of injury, with the ATFL the most commonly injured, followed by the CFL. Cadaveric-sectioning studies have shown that following ATFL rupture, internal rotation forces on the foot increase appreciably, placing the remaining intact ligaments at increased stress.[11] Broström found that combined ruptures of the ATFL and CFL occurred in 20% of cases, whereas isolated CFL rupture was rare.[12] Injury to the PTFL is also rare in ankle sprains, but is more commonly associated with ankle fractures, dislocations, or a combination of the two.[13]

Medial-sided ankle sprains occur much less frequently than those on the lateral side. This is partly because of inversion injuries occurring more frequently but also because of the strength of the medial-sided ligaments. The deltoid ligament is a broad ligament composed of 4 primary components (with 2 more variable components), making it the strongest of the ankle ligaments.[14] Acute medial ankle sprains result from eversion or external rotation forces about the ankle.[15] Usually, landing on an off-balanced pronated foot results in forced external rotation and abduction of the ankle.[14] This typically occurs while walking, running, or jumping on uneven surfaces (**Fig. 4**).[16]

Milner and Soames[17] described what is now the most commonly accepted description of the deltoid ligament. They described 4 superficial and 2 deep components. Superficially, the tibiospring and tibionavicular ligaments are found consistently, whereas there is a variable presence of the superficial tibiotalar and tibiocalcaneal ligaments. These components help align the talus and medial malleolus while resisting external rotation of the talus from under the tibia. They also resist valgus stress of the ankle

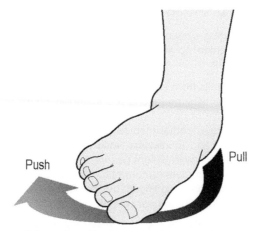

Push   Pull

Fig. 4. Eversion injury of the right ankle. (*From* Hardy M, Snaith B. Musculoskeletal trauma. A guide to assessment and diagnosis. London: Churchill Livingstone; 2011; with permission.)

joint.[18] The deep posterior tibiotalar and the deep anterior tibiotalar ligaments comprise the deeper layer. They also resist lateral displacement and external rotation of the talus, but also serve as the primary stabilizers of the ankle against plantarflexion.[19,20]

High ankle sprains, also known as syndesmotic injuries, involve the distal tibiofibular syndesmosis. They occur less frequently in the general population, but occur commonly in collision sports, including football, ice hockey, and soccer.[21] The injury typically results from an external rotation force applied to the foot in relation to the tibia. Syndesmostic sprains are often associated with further soft tissue injury and fractures, which may lead to significant ankle instability.[22]

The distal tibiofibular syndesmosis consists of the anterior-inferior tibiofibular ligament (AITFL), interosseous ligament, interosseous membrane, posterior-inferior tibiofibular ligament (PITFL), and the inferior transverse ligament. Combined, these tissues serve to prevent dissociation of the tibia and fibula, as well as preventing posterolateral bowing of the fibular during activities that stress the fibula (**Fig. 5**).[23]

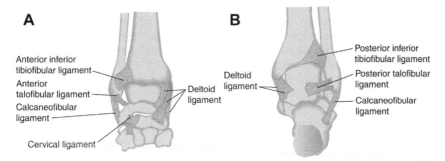

A

Anterior inferior tibiofibular ligament

Anterior talofibular ligament

Calcaneofibular ligament

Cervical ligament

Deltoid ligament

B

Deltoid ligament

Posterior inferior tibiofibular ligament

Posterior talofibular ligament

Calcaneofibular ligament

Fig. 5. Anterior and posterior renderings of the distal tibiotalar syndesmosis. (*From* DeLee JC, Drez D, Miller MD. DeLee and Drez's orthopedic sports medicine. Philadelphia: Saunders; 2010; with permission.)

CLASSIFICATION OF ANKLE SPRAINS

Several grading and staging systems for lateral ankle sprains exist. Kaikkonen and colleagues[24] classified ankle sprains into perhaps the most useful and popular scheme of grades of I to III:

Grade I: mild sprain; results from stretch of ligaments without macroscopic tearing; little swelling or tenderness; no mechanical instability on examination; no loss of function or motion.

Grade II: moderate sprain; partial macroscopic tear of the ligaments; moderate swelling, ecchymosis, and tenderness; mild to moderate instability; some loss of motion; moderate pain with weight bearing and ambulation.

Grade III: severe sprain; complete rupture of the ligaments; severe swelling, ecchymosis, tenderness, and pain; significant mechanical instability; significant loss of function and motion; inability to bear weight.

Clinically, simple sprains (Grade I) will normally not require anything more than symptomatic treatment, whereas more severe sprains (Grades II–III) may require additional treatment.[9]

Hintermann[16] developed a useful classification scheme for medial-sided ankle sprains based on location and severity of injury:

Type I: mild tears or avulsions of the tibionavicular or tibiospring ligaments.

Type II: intermediate tears of the same ligaments.

Type III: distal, more severe tears of the tibionavicular and spring ligaments.

DIAGNOSIS OF ANKLE SPRAINS

Physical examination of the ankle includes careful inspection, palpation, determination of weight-bearing ability, and injury-specific diagnostic maneuvers. First, inspect for swelling and ecchymosis. Palpation should include the entire fibula, distal tibia, the foot, and the Achilles tendon. Significant swelling and pain on palpation is commonly present in patients with ligament rupture. Tenderness over ligamentous structures is a nonspecific finding, but often correlates with structural injury. Tenderness over areas specified by the Ottawa ankle rules may indicate fracture associated with inversion or eversion injuries.[25] These areas include the posterior edge or tip of the lateral malleolus, posterior edge or tip of the medial malleolus, the base of the fifth metatarsal, and the navicular bone. Palpation over the entire fibula is important, especially in syndesmotic injuries, as proximal fibular pain may indicate the eponymous proximal fibular Maisonneuve fracture (**Figs. 6** and **7**).

The presence of swelling, hematoma, localized pain on palpation, and a positive anterior drawer test are indicative of a lateral ankle sprain.[9] A more reliable diagnosis can be made in the subacute period after the initial pain and swelling have subsided. A rupture is rare in the absence of pain on palpation of the ATFL. Alternatively, localized pain on palpation in addition to hematoma discoloration suggests a 90% chance of acute rupture.[26] A positive anterior drawer test is highly sensitive and specific for ATFL injury, and even more so when combined with pain on palpation of the ATFL and presence of hematoma. A positive talar tilt test may indicate a tear that has extended posteriorly to the CFL.[27]

Medial-sided ankle sprains will demonstrate swelling and tenderness at the tip of the medial malleolus, as well as tenderness at the deltoid ligament. The integrity of the superficial deltoid ligament can be assessed with the eversion stress test, whereas the external rotation test can be used to evaluate the deep deltoid ligament and

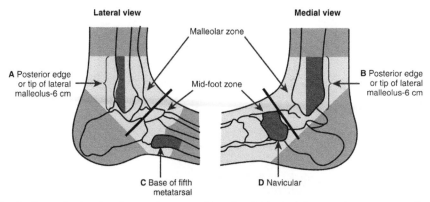

Fig. 6. Sites of palpation for the Ottawa ankle rules. (*Adapted from* Bachmann LM, Kolb E, Koller MT, et al. Accuracy of Ottawa ankle rules to exclude fractures of the ankle and mid-foot; systematic review. BMJ 2003;326:417–9; with permission.)

syndesmosis.[28] The anterior drawer test also may be used to evaluate for anterior and medial subluxation with deltoid ligament injury.[16]

Syndesmotic sprains may have localized pain and tenderness with palpation of the AITFL, PITFL, and medial malleolus. The presence of a widened mortise on radiographic examination indicates a syndesmotic injury as well.

PHYSICAL EXAMINATION TESTS ABOUT THE ANKLE
Anterior Drawer Test

The anterior drawer test assesses for anterior subluxation of the talus from the tibia. Performed by stabilizing the leg with one hand, and with the foot held in neutral position (slightly plantar flexed and inverted), the examiner grasps the heel and applies a gentle and sturdy anterior force at the heel. Instability may be assessed by comparing to the uninjured side; a grossly positive finding indicates rupture of the ATFL (**Fig. 8**).

Talar Tilt Test

The talar tilt test evaluates excessive ankle inversion. With the ankle in neutral position, a gentle inversion force is applied to the ankle and the degree of inversion is noted and compared with the uninjured side; a positive test indicates CFL tear (**Fig. 9**).

A series of ankle x ray films is required only if there is any pain in malleolar zone and any of these findings: • Bone tenderness at **A** • Bone tenderness at **B** • Inability to bear weight both immediately and in emergency department	A series of ankle x ray films is required only if there is any pain in mid-foot zone and any of these findings: • Bone tenderness at **C** • Bone tenderness at **D** • Inability to bear weight both immediately and in emergency department

Fig. 7. Guidelines for ordering ankle series radiographs according to the Ottawa ankle rules. (*Adapted from* Bachmann LM, Kolb E, Koller MT, et al. Accuracy of Ottawa ankle rules to exclude fractures of the ankle and mid-foot; systematic review. BMJ 2003;326:417–9; with permission.)

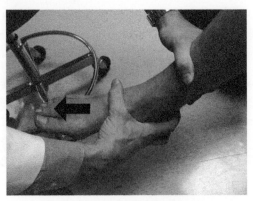

Fig. 8. Anterior drawer test. (*From* Hurt J. Physical examination and evaluation. In: Johnson DL, Mair SD, editors. Clinical sports medicine. Philadelphia: Elsevier; with permission.)

Eversion Stress Test

The eversion stress test is performed with the patient's leg dangling from the examination table. The leg is stabilized with one hand while the other hand grasps the calcaneus applying an eversion stress by rolling the calcaneus laterally; pain indicates a deltoid ligament injury.

External Rotation Test

The external rotation test is performed with the knee flexed at 90° and the ankle in neutral position. The examiner stabilizes the leg proximal to the ankle joint with one hand while the other hand grasps the plantar aspect of the foot and externally rotates the foot; pain indicates a syndesmotic sprain (**Fig. 10**).

Squeeze Test

In the squeeze test, the leg is gently compressed from the medial and lateral sides at the mid-calf level; pain indicates a syndesmotic injury (**Fig. 11**).

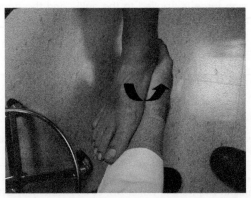

Fig. 9. Talar tilt test. (*From* Hurt J. Physical examination and evaluation. In: Johnson DL, Mair SD, editors. Clinical sports medicine. Philadelphia: Elsevier; with permission.)

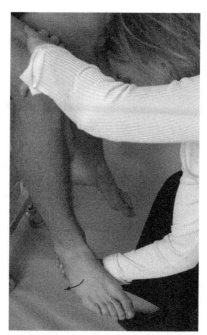

Fig. 10. External rotation test. (*From* Magee D. Orthopedic physical assessment. Philadelphia: Saunders; 2008; with permission.)

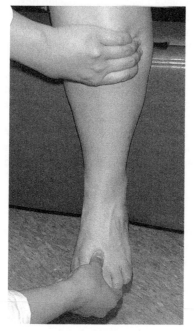

Fig. 11. Squeeze test. (*From* Lee TK, Maleski R. Physical examination of the ankle for ankle pathology. Clin Podiatr Med Sur 2002;19(2):251–69; with permission.)

GUIDELINES FOR OBTAINING ANKLE RADIOGRAPHS

Stiell and colleagues[25] developed the "Ottawa ankle rules," a set of guidelines used to indicate the need for standard ankle radiographs to exclude fractures and associated pathology (see **Figs. 6** and **7**). Tenderness to palpation of specific areas about the ankle joint and an inability to bear weight indicate the need for radiographic studies. Fractures should be referred to orthopedic surgery.

TREATMENT OF ACUTE ANKLE SPRAINS

The treatment of acute ankle sprains involves 2 stages: (1) acute and (2) early mobilization with gradual rehabilitation. Acute treatment focuses on minimizing swelling in and around the ankle joint, control of pain, protection from further injury, promotion of healing, and initiation of rehabilitation to limit long-term deficits in strength, flexibility, and endurance. The goals of early mobilization with rehabilitation include restoration of range of motion (especially dorsiflexion), restoration of strength (especially the peroneal muscles), restoration of proprioception, and safe return to activity. Acute treatment begins after initial injury and continues until pain and swelling resolve. A mnemonic used to remember the essential components of acute treatment is PRICEMMMS, an extension of RICE.[29]

Protection from further injury. An aircast can be used to restrict the inversion and eversion stress on the injured ankle, while maintaining dorsiflexion and plantarflexion. It should be used continuously until swelling, strength deficits, and flexibility deficits resolve. Then its use may be limited to during exercise.

Rest.

Ice is effective as long as swelling is present.[30] A bag of crushed ice should be placed directly on the skin for 20 minutes every hour.

Compression may be achieved with a compression hose or wrap. Direct compression helps to promote resorption of edema out of the joint space, which allows for earlier range of motion and mobility.[31]

Elevation above the level of the heart will improve venous return and decrease swelling.[32]

Medications, such as analgesics and nonsteroidal anti-inflammatories, have an important role in controlling pain and inflammation after acute injury.

Modalities such as electrical muscle stimulation can be used to control pain, and maintain muscle strength and range of motion.

Mobilization should begin on the day the injury occurs. Active plantarflexion and dorsiflexion limited to a pain-free range of motion can improve edema mobilization.

Strength training of the peroneal and gastrocnemius muscles also should begin as soon as possible.

REHABILITATION

Rehabilitation is an important component of treatment of acute ankle sprains. Regaining normal function and strength of the ankle, and preventing future reinjury are the primary goals of rehabilitation. It is important to implement a program that introduces exercises at higher levels of stress to the ankle in a stepwise fashion. Although it may be tempting for patients to return to normal physical activities after resolution of pain and swelling, lack of proper rehabilitation places the patient at risk for recurrent, more severe ankle injury with potential to develop into chronic functional instability.

Activities such as strength training, water jogging, swimming, and cycling help to improve strength, range of motion, and proprioception while maintaining cardiovascular fitness. This ensures that when the ankle is fully rehabilitated, the cardiovascular fitness of the patient is adequate to resume normal activities. Range of motion exercises include "ankle pumps" (ie, plantarflexion and dorsiflexion) and inversion/eversion motions. Resistance exercise bands may also be incorporated into the rehabilitation exercises as soon as they can be performed pain free.

After full rehabilitation, patients may return to physical activity and sports progressively. An athlete should begin with simple drills and progress to no restrictions. The use of a brace should continue until the athlete is cleared to play without restrictions. A brace allows for improved proprioceptive feedback during exercise.[33,34]

COMMON THERAPEUTIC MODALITIES
Ultrasound

- No difference in general improvement in symptoms or functional disability between ultrasound and sham ultrasound after 7 days.
- After 14 days, however, those treated with ultrasound showed a significant improvement compared with immobilization.[35]

Contrast Bath

- Alternating warm and cold water helps stimulate peripheral circulation and may decrease edema.

Electrical Stimulation

- Transcutaneous electrical neuromuscular stimulator (TENS) is a biphasic current that stimulates sensory nerves to mitigate pain-signaling pathway and stimulate endorphin production to normalize sympathetic function.

Massage

- Retrograde massage techniques may help to reduce swelling by compressing edematous fluid intravascularly.

Taping

- Improves proprioception due to sensory input from pressure on the skin; also reduces swelling via compression while maintaining an element of immobilization.[36]

ANKLE INSTABILITY

Acute ankle sprains may lead to mechanical or functional deficits resulting in chronic ankle instability.[37]

Mechanical causes of chronic instability may include the following:

- Pathologic laxity
- Arthrokinetic restriction
- Synovial changes
- Degenerative changes

Functional causes of chronic instability may include the following:

- Proprioception abnormalities
- Neuromuscular control loss
- Postural control impairment
- Strength deficits

Patients suffering from ankle instability will complain of persistent pain and repeated instances of their ankle giving way, often partly due to increased ankle joint laxity. However, chronic ankle instability may be present without increased ligamentous laxity.[38]

Degenerative joint changes about the ankle may be the cause or effect of chronic ankle instability. Such intra-articular pathology includes the following:

- Osteochondral lesions of the talus
- Impingement
- Loose bodies
- Painful ossicles
- Adhesions
- Chondromalacia
- Osteophytes

These degenerative changes have a higher incidence of occurring on the medial side of the ankle.[39] Upwards of two-thirds of patients with chronic ankle instability will present with a predominance of medial-sided articular injuries according to one study.[40]

TREATING CHRONIC ANKLE INSTABILITY

The first line of treatment for chronic ankle stability includes neuromuscular training. This consists of exercises intended to improve strength and balance and often leads to full functional recovery. Specifically, the goal is to optimize lower limb postural control and restore active stability. These exercises include the following:

- "Wobble board" activities[41]
- "Hop to stabilization" exercises[42]
- Single-limb stance balance activities[43]

Additionally, taping or bracing the affected ankle can provide extra mechanical support and improved proprioception.[36,43] Several ankle-foot orthoses are available depending on the cause and nature of the instability.

SURGICAL OPTIONS

Various surgical procedures aim to provide stability when conservative treatment fails, which often occurs. Surgical treatment of chronic ankle instability is either via anatomic repair or tenodesis stabilization.

Common anatomic repairs include the following:

- Broström technique: midsubstance imbrication and suture of the lateral ankle ligaments.[44]
- Gould augmentation: augmentation of the Broström repair with mobilized lateral portion of the extensor retinaculum.[45]
- Karlsson technique: anchoring the proximal ligament ends through drill holes (**Fig. 12**).[46]

Common tenodesis stabilization procedures include the following:

- Watson-Jones procedure: peroneus brevis graft tenodesis to fibula and talus.[47]
- Evans procedure: peroneus brevis graft tenodesis to fibula.[48]
- Chrisman-Snook procedure: split peroneus brevis graft tenodesis to fibula and calcaneus (**Fig. 13**).[49]

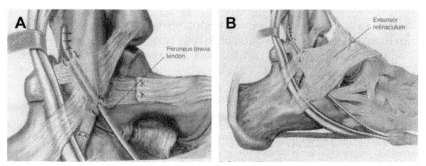

Fig. 12. Illustration demonstrating anatomic repairs of chronic lateral ankle instability. (*A*) Broström technique. (*B*) Gould modification. (*Adapted from* Gerard P. Clinical evaluation of the modified Brostrom-Evans procedure to restore ankle stability. Foot Ankle Int 1999;20:246–52; with permission.)

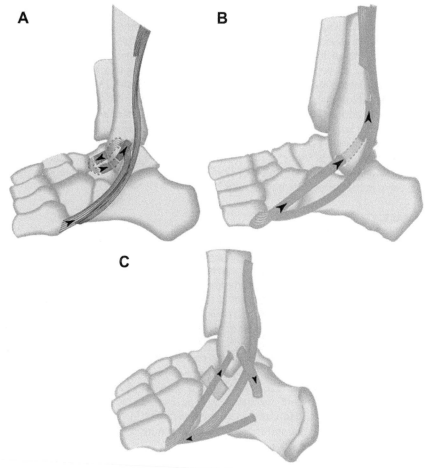

Fig. 13. Illustration demonstrating tenodesis reconstruction for chronic lateral ankle instability. (*A*) Watson-Jones procedure. (*B*) Evans procedure. (*C*) Chrisman-Snook procedure. (*From* DeLee JC, Drez D, Miller MD. DeLee and Drez's orthopedic sports medicine. Philadelphia: Saunders; 2010; with permission.)

Several outcome studies have been done to compare the various techniques. Generally, the Broström procedure and its modifications have been very successful with few complications.[50] One long-term retrospective study demonstrated anatomic reconstruction procedures had better overall results than certain tenodesis procedures.[51]

TREATMENT RECOMMENDATIONS REMAIN INCONCLUSIVE

The spectrum of treatment for ankle sprains and instability includes initial immobilization with cast or splint, functional treatment comprising early immobilization and use of an external support (eg, ankle brace), and surgical repair or reconstruction. Several studies have compared nonoperative with surgical treatment for injuries to the ligamentous complex about the ankle. One such meta-analysis includes 20 trials involving 2562 mostly young active adult males.[52] Although certain analytic models favor surgical treatment for the 4 primary outcomes (return to preinjury level of sprains, ankle sprain recurrence, long-term pain, subjective or functional instability), the investigators conclude insufficient evidence exists from randomized controlled trials to determine the relative effectiveness of surgical versus conservative treatment. Another meta-analysis demonstrated that after surgical reconstruction, early functional rehabilitation was shown to be superior to 6 weeks of immobilization regarding time to return to work and sports.[53] This review of 7 randomized trials, however, also concludes insufficient evidence exists to support any specific surgical or conservative intervention for chronic ankle instability. While looking specifically at athletes, 1 review concluded early functional treatment provided the fastest recovery of ankle mobility and earliest return to work and physical activity without affecting late mechanical stability. Functional treatment was complication-free, whereas surgery had serious, although infrequent, complications. Functional treatment produced no more sequelae than casting with or without surgical repair. Secondary surgical repair, even years after an injury, has results comparable with those of primary repair, so even competitive athletes can receive initial conservative treatment.[54]

SUMMARY

Ankle sprains are among the most common musculoskeletal injuries presenting to emergency departments and primary care providers within the United States, especially among teenagers, young adults, and athletes. Most ankle sprains are inversion injuries to the lateral ligamentous complex, although medial-sided and high ankle sprains also represent injuries that should be recognized. Providers should obtain a detailed history and perform a thorough physical examination to delineate the location and extent of injury. Providers should apply the Ottawa ankle rules to determine when radiography is indicated and refer fractures and more severe injuries to orthopedic surgery as needed. Acute sprains should be comprehensively treated with previously well-described conservative measures, with providers bearing in mind that previous ankle sprain poses the greatest risk for future sprains and a greater likelihood of chronic instability. Treatment for these injuries remains somewhat controversial. Low-grade injuries have been shown to respond well to nonoperative treatment, whereas high-grade injuries and those chronic in nature may require surgical treatment in addition to conservative measures.

REFERENCES

1. Boruta PM, Bishop JO, Braly WG, et al. Acute lateral ankle ligament injuries: a literature review. Foot Ankle 1990;11(2):107–13.

2. Waterman BR, Owens BD, Davey S, et al. The epidemiology of ankle sprains in the United States. J Bone Joint Surg Am 2010;92(13):2279–84.

3. Soboroff SH, Pappius EM, Komaroff AL. Benefits, risks, and costs of alternative approaches to the evaluation and treatment of severe ankle sprain. Clin Orthop Relat Res 1984;183:160–8.

4. Gerber JP, Williams GN, Scoville CR, et al. Persistent disability associated with ankle sprains: a prospective examination of an athletic population. Foot Ankle Int 1998;19:653–60.

5. Yeung MS, Chan KM, So CH, et al. An epidemiological survey on ankle sprain. Br J Sports Med 1994;28:112–6.

6. Anandacoomarasamy A, Barnsley L. Long-term outcomes of inversion ankle injuries. Br J Sports Med 2005;39:e14 [discussion: e14].

7. McKay GD, Goldie PA, Payne WR, et al. Ankle injuries in basketball: injury rate and risk factors. Br J Sports Med 2001;35(2):103–8.

8. Tiemstra JD. Update on acute ankle sprains. Am Fam Physician 2012;85(12): 1170–6.

9. van den Bekerom MP, Kerkhoffs GM, McColum GA, et al. Management of acute lateral ankle ligament injury in the athlete. Knee Surg Sports Traumatol Arthrosc 2013;21(6):1390–5.

10. Garrick JG. The frequency of injury, mechanism of injury, and epidemiology of ankle sprains. Am J Sports Med 1977;5:241–2.

11. Kjaersgaard-Andersen P, Wethelund JO, Helmig P, et al. The stabilizing effect of the ligamentous structures in the sinus and canalis tarsi on movements in the hindfoot: an experimental study. Am J Sports Med 1988;16: 512–6.

12. Broström L. Sprained ankles. V. Treatment and prognosis in recent ligament ruptures. Acta Chir Scand 1966;132(5):537–50.

13. Safran MR, Benedetti RS, Bartolozzi AR III, et al. Lateral ankle sprains: a comprehensive review: part I: etiology, pathoanatomy, histopathogenesis, and diagnosis. Med Sci Sports Exerc 1999;31(Suppl 7):429–37.

14. Savage-Elliott I, Murawski CD, Smyth NA, et al. The deltoid ligament: an in-depth review of anatomy, function, and treatment strategies. Knee Surg Sports Traumatol Arthrosc 2012;21(6):1316–27.

15. O'Loughlin P, Murawski CD, Egan C, et al. Ankle instability in sports. Phys Sportsmed 2009;37(2):1–12.

16. Hintermann B. Medial ankle instability. Foot Ankle Clin 2003;8(4):723–38.

17. Milner CE, Soames RW. Anatomy of the collateral ligaments of the human ankle joint. Foot Ankle 1998;19(11):757–60.

18. Beals TC, Crim J, Nickisch F. Deltoid ligament injuries in athletes: techniques of repair and reconstruction. Oper Tech Sports Med 2010;18(1):11–7.

19. Jelinek JA, Porter DA. Management of unstable ankle fractures and syndesmosis injuries in athletes. Foot Ankle Clin 2009;14(2):277–98.

20. Michelson JD, Waldman B. An axially loaded model of the ankle after pronation external rotation injury. Clin Orthop Relat Res 1996;328:285–93.

21. Boytim MJ, Fischer DA, Neumann L. Syndesmotic ankle sprains. Am J Sports Med 1991;19:294–8.

22. Zalavras C, Thordarson D. Ankle syndesmotic injury. J Am Acad Orthop Surg 2007;15:330–9.

23. Thomas KA, Harris MB, Willis MC, et al. The effects of the interosseous membrane and partial fibulectomy on loading of the tibia: a biomechanical study. Orthopedics 1995;18:373–83.

24. Kaikkonen A, Kannus P, Jarvinen M. A performance test protocol and scoring scale for the evaluation of ankle injuries. Am J Sports Med 1994;22(4):462–9.

25. Stiell IG, Greenberg GH, McKnight RD, et al. A study to develop clinical decision rules for the use of radiography in acute ankle injuries. Ann Emerg Med 1992;21(4):384–90.

26. Van Dijk CN, Mol BW, Lim LS, et al. Diagnosis of ligament rupture of the ankle joint. Physical examination, arthrography, stress radiography and sonography compared in 160 patients after inversion trauma. Acta Orthop Scand 1996; 67(6):566–70.

27. Hintermann B, Valderrabano V. Medial ankle/deltoid ligament reconstruction. In: Easley ME, Wiesel SW, editors. Operative technique of the foot and ankle. Philadelphia: Lippincott Williams & Wilkins; 2010. p. 874–86.

28. Lynch SA. Assessment of the injured ankle in the athlete. J Athl Train 2002;37: 406–12.

29. Chorley JN, Hergenroeder AC. Management of ankle sprains. Pediatr Ann 1997; 26(1):56–64.

30. Basur RL, Shephard E, Mouzas GL. A cooling method in the treatment of ankle sprains. Practitioner 1976;216(1296):708–11.

31. Wilkerson GB, Horn-Kingery HM. Treatment of the inversion ankle sprain: comparison of different modes of compression and cryotherapy. J Orthop Sports Phys Ther 1993;17:240–6.

32. Sims D. Effects of positioning on ankle edema. J Orthop Sports Phys Ther 1986; 8:30–4.

33. Carroll MJ, Rijke AM, Perrin DH. Effect of the Swede-O ankle brace on talar tilt in subjects with unstable ankles. J Sport Rehabil 1993;2:261–7.

34. Feuerbach JW, Grabiner MD. Effect of the aircast on unilateral postural control: amplitude and frequency variables. J Orthop Sports Phys Ther 1993;17:149–54.

35. Struijs P, Kerkhoffs G. Ankle sprain. Clin Evid 2007;12:1115.

36. Robbins S, Waked E, Rappel R. Ankle taping improves proprioception before and after exercise in young men. Br J Sports Med 1995;29(4):242–7.

37. Hertel J. Functional anatomy, pathomechanics, and pathophysiology of lateral ankle instability. J Athl Train 2002;37:364–75.

38. Bozkurt M, Doral MN. Anatomic factors and biomechanics in ankle instability. Foot Ankle Clin 2006;11(3):451–63.

39. Harrington KD. Degenerative arthritis of the ankle secondary to long-standing lateral ligament instability. J Bone Joint Surg Am 1979;61(3):354–61.

40. Van Dijk CN, Bossuyt PM, Marti RK, et al. Medial ankle pain after lateral ligament rupture. J Bone Joint Surg Br 1996;78(4):562–7.

41. Clark VM, Burden AM. A 4-week wobble board exercise programme improved muscle onset latency and perceived stability in individuals with a functionally unstable ankle. Phys Ther Sport 2005;6(4):181–7.

42. McKeon PO, Ingersoll CD, Kerrigan DC, et al. Balance training improves function and postural control in those with chronic ankle instability. Med Sci Sports Exerc 2008;40(10):1810–9.

43. Baier M, Hopf T. Ankle orthoses effect on single-limb standing balance in athletes with functional ankle instability. Arch Phys Med Rehabil 1998;79(8): 939–44.

44. Broström L. Sprained ankles: VI Surgical treatment of "chronic" ligament ruptures. Acta Chir Scand 1966;132:551–65.

45. Gould N, Seligson D, Gassman J, et al. Early and late repair of lateral ligament of the ankle. Foot Ankle 1980;1:84–9.

46. Karlsson J, Bergsten T, Lansinger O, et al. Lateral ankle instability of the ankle treated by the Evans procedure: a long-term clinical and radiological follow-up. J Bone Joint Surg Br 1988;70:476–80.
47. Watson-Jones R. Recurrent forward dislocation of the ankle joint. J Bone Joint Surg Br 1952;143:519.
48. Evans DL. Recurrent instability of the ankle: a method of surgical treatment. Proc R Soc Med 1953;46:343–4.
49. Chrisman OD, Snook GA. Reconstruction of lateral ligament tears of the ankle: an experimental study and clinical evaluation of seven patients treated by a new modification of the Elmslie procedure. J Bone Joint Surg Am 1969;51:904–12.
50. Hennrikus WL, Mapes RC, Lyons PM, et al. Outcomes of the Chrisman-Snook and modified-Brostrom procedures for chronic lateral ankle instability: a prospective, randomized comparison. Am J Sports Med 1996;24:400–4.
51. Krips R, Brandsson S, Swensson C, et al. Anatomical reconstruction and Evans tenodesis of the lateral ligaments of the ankle: clinical and radiological findings after follow-up for 15 to 30 years. J Bone Joint Surg Br 2002;84:232–6.
52. Kerkhoffs GM, Handoll HH, de Bie R, et al. Surgical versus conservative treatment for acute injuries of the lateral ligament complex of the ankle in adults. Cochrane Database Syst Rev 2007;(2):CD000380.
53. de Vries JS, Krips R, Sierevelt IN, et al. Interventions for treating chronic ankle instability. Cochrane Database Syst Rev 2011;(8):CD004124.
54. Lynch SA, Renström PA. Treatment of acute lateral ankle ligament rupture in the athlete. Conservative versus surgical treatment. Sports Med 1999;27(1):61–71.

Achilles Tendon Disorders

Steven B. Weinfeld, MD

KEYWORDS

- Achilles tendon • Retrocalcaneal bursitis • Achilles rupture • Tendinitis
- Achilles tendinosis • Haglund deformity • Paratenonitis

KEY POINTS

- Achilles tendon disorders include tendinosis, paratenonitis, insertional tendinitis, retrocalcaneal bursitis, and frank rupture.
- Patients present with pain and swelling in the posterior aspect of the ankle.
- Magnetic resonance imaging and ultrasound are helpful for confirming the diagnosis and guiding treatment.
- Nonsurgical management of Achilles tendon disorders includes nonsteroidal anti-inflammatory drugs, physical therapy, bracing, and footwear modification.
- Surgical treatment includes debridement of the diseased area of the tendon with direct repair.
- Tendon transfer may be necessary to augment the strength of the Achilles tendon.

INTRODUCTION

Disorders of the Achilles tendon can occur in adolescents and adults, and include both traumatic and nontraumatic problems, such as insertional tendinitis, intra-substance tendinopathy, and complete rupture. Paratenonitis and retrocalcaneal bursitis also cause pain around the Achilles tendon. Symptoms include swelling and pain in the posterior aspect of the ankle or heel. Diagnosis can be confirmed with imaging, including ultrasound and magnetic resonance imaging (MRI). Treatment consists of nonsurgical measures, including ice, nonsteroidal anti-inflammatory drugs (NSAIDs), heel lifts, immobilization, and physical therapy. Surgical treatment is indicated when conservative measures have not relieved symptoms, and includes tendon debridement and repair, resection of bony prominences, and tendon transfer.

ACHILLES TENDON ANATOMY

The Achilles tendon is formed by the gastrocnemius and soleus muscles at their attachment to the posterior aspect of the calcaneus. The Achilles tendon does not

Foot and Ankle Service, Icahn School of Medicine at Mount Sinai, New York, NY, USA
E-mail address: steven.weinfeld@mountsinai.org

Med Clin N Am 98 (2014) 331–338
http://dx.doi.org/10.1016/j.mcna.2013.11.005   medical.theclinics.com
0025-7125/14/$ – see front matter © 2014 Elsevier Inc. All rights reserved.

have a true synovial sheath, but rather a single layer of paratenon. This paratenon is a single layer of cells composed of fatty areolar tissue that is highly vascularized. The paratenon is responsible for a significant portion of the blood supply to the Achilles tendon. Most of the blood supply to the Achilles enters anteriorly, and studies have shown a hypovascular area 2 to 6 cm proximal to the insertion on the calcaneus.[1]

Imaging

The Achilles tendon is best imaged using ultrasonography and MRI. Ultrasound is fast, safe, and inexpensive and can easily help localize diseased segments of the tendon. In acute Achilles tendinopathy, ultrasound can clearly demonstrate fluid around the tendon. Tendon swelling and thickening, discontinuity of tendon fibers, and focal hypoechoic intratendinous areas are the most common ultrasonic findings in patients with Achilles tendon abnormalities.[2] Ultrasound has some limitations, including the differentiation of a partial Achilles rupture from a discrete area of tendinosis. It is user-dependent and may not be able to distinguish between Achilles tendinosis and paratenonitis. MRI is an excellent technique for imaging the internal morphology of the Achilles tendon. It can easily distinguish between paratenonitis and tendinosis. MRI is not user-dependent and can provide multiplanar images of the Achilles. It is also useful in determining the extent of degeneration in the tendon, which is useful for preoperative planning.[3]

INSERTIONAL ACHILLES TENDINITIS

Insertional Achilles tendon problems occur at the Achilles attachment site on the posterior aspect of the calcaneus. Degeneration of the tendon and varying degrees of calcification at the insertion site are present. Insertional Achilles tendonitis is usually atraumatic in onset and occurs in older patients.

Diagnosis

Patients with insertional Achilles tendinitis complain of pain at the posterior aspect of the heel. A bony prominence or Haglund deformity is often present.[4] Difficulty with footwear is common. Patients usually report pain and stiffness on arising after sleep or after sitting for some time. A shoe with a raised heel is often more comfortable than a flat shoe. Examination reveals tenderness at the insertion of the Achilles accompanied by swelling and a bony prominence. Thickening of the Achilles tendon may be present with more chronic inflammation. Some pain may be elicited with passive dorsiflexion of the foot. Radiographs are helpful in determining the presence of a bony Haglund deformity at the posterior aspect of the calcaneus. MRI can be helpful in determining the extent of the degeneration of the Achilles tendon.

Treatment

Treatment of insertional Achilles tendinitis includes anti-inflammatory medication and footwear modification. Heel lifts may alleviate pain by elevating the heel to reduce tension on the Achilles insertion. The heel lift may also decrease shoe irritation over the bony prominence posteriorly. Immobilization with a boot brace or cast may be necessary in patients who do not improve with other measures. Physical therapy, including Achilles tendon stretching, may also be helpful to reduce inflammation and pain. Surgery is indicated when conservative therapy is not beneficial.

Surgical Treatment

Surgery for insertional Achilles tendon problems should include debridement of the degenerated tendon and resection of the bony deformity. In some cases of severe tendinosis, a tendon transfer may be necessary to restore adequate plantarflexion strength. Most authors recommend a tendon transfer if greater than 50% of the Achilles tendon is diseased.[5] This procedure is usually performed using the flexor hallucis longus tendon. A central tendon splitting approach is used most often to allow adequate debridement of degenerated tendon and resection of calcific densities or bone.[4] The retrocalcaneal bursa is often removed to prevent recurrent pain in this area.

Postoperative Care

After surgery for repair of insertional Achilles tendinitis, a cast is usually required for 6 weeks to protect the tendon-bone interface and to ensure proper anchoring of the tendon. Patients then are placed into a removable boot brace for approximately 1 month and begin physical therapy to restore range of motion and strength. Patients should be informed that full recovery after surgical repair of the Achilles tendon can require up to 12 months.

ACHILLES TENDINOSIS

Degeneration of the Achilles tendon within its midsubstance is very common. On gross examination, Achilles tendinosis appears as a yellowish, thickened tendon from accumulation of mucinous material within the diseased area. This condition can occur in runners and patients with systemic diseases such as lupus or rheumatoid arthritis. Fluoroquinolone antibiotics have also been implicated as a cause of tendinopathy of the Achilles.[6] Systemic factors, including hypertension and hormone replacement therapy, are causes of tendinopathy in women, whereas obesity is an etiologic factor in both men and women because of diminished local vascularity. Foot pronation has been proposed as a mechanical cause of Achilles tendinopathy.[7]

Diagnosis

Achilles tendinopathy presents with thickening of the Achilles tendon 5 to 8 cm proximal to the insertion on the calcaneus. Most patients report an insidious onset without trauma. Swelling often accompanies the thickened tendon, with tenderness to palpation over the affected area. Patients complain of pain on arising after sleep or after sitting for extended periods. Walking stairs are also difficult in this population. Tendinosis can also occur as a painless thickening of the Achilles tendon. On ultrasonography, Achilles tendinosis appears as a hypoechoic lesion with or without intratendinous calcification. MRI is also useful in determining the extent of intratendinous degeneration.[8]

Treatment

Nonsurgical treatment of Achilles tendinopathy includes immobilization in a cast or boot brace. Rest, NSAIDs, and ice are also helpful to reduce pain and inflammation. Physical therapy with modalities may also be helpful. Full-length semirigid orthotics can be used to correct excessive pronation. Cortisone injections should be avoided because they could precipitate a frank rupture. Platelet-rich plasma injections have shown some promise in treating Achilles tendinopathy, although more research is needed to establish efficacy.[9] Heel lifts may also provide some symptomatic relief.

Surgical Treatment

Surgery for Achilles tendinopathy is indicated in patients who are refractory to nonsurgical treatment. Surgery includes debridement of the diseased portion of the tendon and suturing of the remaining tendon with absorbable suture. If greater than 50% of the tendon is debrided, augmentation with a flexor hallucis longus tendon transfer is recommended.[10] Allograft reconstruction has also been used in cases of severe tendon degeneration.[11]

Postoperative Care

After surgical treatment of Achilles tendinosis, the affected limb is protected in a cast or boot brace. Those patients requiring tendon transfer or allograft reconstructions will usually need a short leg cast for 6 weeks, followed by progressive weight-bearing in a cam walker brace and physical therapy.

PARATENONITIS

Inflammation of the tissue surrounding the Achilles tendon is referred to as *paratenonitis* and is most common in younger distance runners. Often paratenonitis occurs in conjunction with Achilles tendinosis; however, inflammation of the paratenon can occur in isolation. Histologically, capillary proliferation and inflammatory cells are present within the paratendinous tissue. Myofibroblasts in the paratendinous tissue synthesize collagen in response to stress, leading to constriction of the paratenon and diminution of the blood supply to the Achilles tendon.[12]

Diagnosis

Physical examination will reveal tenderness and swelling both medial and lateral to the Achilles tendon. Patients will often present with tightness of the gastrocnemius-soleus complex. The Silfverskiold test is used to determine the presence of gastrocnemius tightness. In a patient with gastrocnemius tightness, ankle dorsiflexion will increase with the ipsilateral knee flexed compared with the knee extended. The tenderness and thickness will remain fixed with ankle motion in isolated paratenonitis.[13] As the process progresses, the tendon itself becomes thickened in a fusiform shape. Ultrasound can show fluid surrounding the tendon acutely, and adhesions around the tendon with more chronic inflammation. MRI will show thickening of the paratenon, with high signal present on T2-weighted images.

Treatment

Nonsurgical treatment for paratenonitis includes immobilization with a boot brace or solid ankle/foot orthosis. NSAIDs, ice, and physical therapy are also helpful. Younger, more active patients will benefit from activity modification along with a cushioned heel lift or shock-absorbing orthotic in their running shoes. Brisement can be used to help break up adhesions in the paratenon. This procedure is performed by slowly injecting 5 to 10 mL of either lidocaine or saline into the paratenon sheath. Ultrasound is helpful to avoid intratendinous injection.[14]

Surgical Treatment

Surgery is infrequently required in cases of pure paratenonitis and consists of debridement of the adherent paratenon from the posterior, medial, and lateral aspects of the Achilles tendon. The anterior portion of the paratenon is avoided to prevent disruption of the blood supply to the tendon. This procedure can be performed using either open surgery or arthroscopic technique.[10]

Postoperative Care

In cases of isolated paratenon debridement, immediate range of motion is begun to prevent adhesion from scarring. Weight-bearing is permitted in a removable boot brace for the first 3 to 4 weeks postoperatively. Physical therapy begins as soon as wound healing has occurred to optimize range of motion and strength.

RETROCALCANEAL BURSITIS

Retrocalcaneal bursitis is a distinct entity involving inflammation of the retrocalcaneal bursa anterior to the Achilles tendon. The anterior surface of the bursa is composed of fibrocartilage, and the posterior aspect merges with the anterior Achilles paratenon. The bursa can become hypertrophied and inflamed, resulting in adhesion to the Achilles tendon, which causes degenerative changes within the tendon. This inflammation often occurs in conjunction with a Haglund deformity, with the bursa being compressed with ankle dorsiflexion.[15]

Diagnosis

Tenderness just anterior to the Achilles tendon at the level of insertion is present in patients with retrocalcaneal bursitis. Medial and lateral compression will elicit pain in the posterior aspect of the ankle. Plain radiographs are useful to rule out a bony prominence in the affected area. Ultrasound and MRI are used to determine the presence of inflammatory fluid anterior to the Achilles tendon and any associated degeneration of the tendon or ossification.

Treatment

NSAIDs, activity modification, and bracing are the mainstays of treatment for retrocalcaneal bursitis. Cortisone injection should be avoided to prevent frank rupture of the Achilles tendon. Surgery to remove the bursa and any associated bony prominence is rarely necessary.

Surgical Treatment

Occasionally surgical treatment is required to remove the inflamed bursa and associated bony prominence. This removal can be performed through open surgery and endoscopic technique.[16] Postoperative management is similar to that for other Achilles tendon procedures.

ACHILLES RUPTURE

Complete rupture of the Achilles tendon usually occurs as a result of a sudden contraction of the gastrocnemius-soleus muscle complex. It most often occurs during sports such as tennis, basketball, soccer, and badminton, but can also occur with sudden dorsiflexion of the foot. Patients describe the feeling of being struck in the back of the leg; however, this is rarely the cause. Patients are usually unable to walk immediately after rupture of the Achilles. Achilles rupture can also occur as a result of corticosteroid use.[6] Extreme caution should be used when injecting steroids near the Achilles tendon.[17]

Diagnosis

Achilles rupture is often suspected based on the history of the injury. Physical examination reveals a palpable gap in the Achilles tendon. The most frequent site of rupture is approximately 6 cm proximal to the insertion of the tendon on the calcaneus. The

Thompson test is positive with a complete Achilles tendon rupture (**Fig. 1**). Imaging is not usually necessary if the Thompson test is positive and a palpable gap is present.[18] If a calcaneal avulsion fracture is suspected, radiographs should be obtained. MRI can help confirm the diagnosis. Ultrasound may also be a helpful diagnostic modality.

Treatment

Clinical studies support both nonsurgical treatment with immobilization and surgical repair for Achilles rupture. Most studies report a slightly lower rerupture rate with surgical repair.[19] Wound complications are common with surgery. Achilles ruptures can be immobilized with casts or braces. Care should be taken to ensure that the torn ends of the tendon are closely apposed in the brace or cast. Ultrasound has been shown to be helpful for confirming apposition of the tendon ends in patients treated with bracing. Surgical repair is performed using either open technique or percutaneous methods.[20] Injury to the sural nerve should be avoided. Deep venous thrombosis is not infrequent with Achilles rupture. Some evidence supports anticoagulation therapy in patients with Achilles ruptures.[21]

Postoperative Treatment

After repair of a ruptured Achilles tendon, a splint or cast is applied with the foot in slight plantarflexion. Patients remain non–weight-bearing on the affected limb for 4 weeks and progress from a cast to a boot brace during that period. Physical therapy begins at 6 weeks postoperatively to restore range of motion and strength. A half-inch heel lift is recommended for approximately 6 months once the patient has returned to regular shoes. Return to sports often requires a minimum of 6 to 9 months. Most patients will require 12 to 18 months for full restoration of strength.

CHRONIC ACHILLES RUPTURE

A chronic rupture is defined as a rupture neglected for more than 4 weeks.[22] Patients usually recall some pain and swelling in the posterior ankle. These ruptures typically occur 3 to 6 cm proximal to the calcaneal insertion. Patients will complain of difficulty with push off of the affected limb. Examination reveals thickening of the Achilles tendon in the region of injury. The Thompson test may be positive, indicating a nonfunctional tendon. A palpable gap may be present with varying degrees of

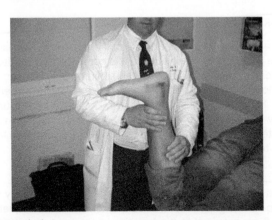

Fig. 1. The Thompson test.

tenderness, depending on the chronicity of the rupture. Patients will be unable to perform a single heel rise, indicating significant weakness of the gastrocnemius-soleus complex.

Treatment

The goal of treatment in a chronic Achilles tendon rupture is to adequately restore the optimal length and continuity of the gastrocnemius-soleus complex. How this is accomplished depends on the size of the defect in the tendon. With gaps of up to 4 cm, end-to-end tendon repair is usually possible.[22] In larger defects, a V-Y advancement procedure or turndown of the central slip is used to restore the integrity of the tendon. Most authors recommend flexor tendon augmentation in conjunction with a V-Y advancement or central turndown.[23,24] This approach is usually performed using a flexor hallucis longus tendon transfer. Synthetic materials and collagen allografts are also available to augment the tendon repair.[25] Achilles allografts have been used to reconstruct very large defects, usually greater than 10 cm.[11]

REFERENCES

1. Chen TM, Rozen WM, Pan WR, et al. The arterial anatomy of the Achilles tendon: anatomical study and clinical implications. Clin Anat 2009;22(3):377–85.
2. Paavola M, Paakkala T, Kannus P, et al. Ultrasonography in the differential diagnosis of Achilles tendon injuries and related disorders: a comparison between pre-operative ultrasonography and surgical findings. Acta Radiol 1998; 39:612–9.
3. Goodwin DW. Imaging of the Achilles tendon. Foot Ankle Clin 2000;5(1):135–48.
4. McGarvey WC, Palumbo RC, Baxter DE, et al. Insertional Achilles tendinosis: surgical treatment through a central tendon splitting approach. Foot Ankle Int 2002; 23:19–25.
5. Den Hartog BD. Flexor hallucis longus transfer for chronic Achilles tendinosis. Foot Ankle Int 2003;24:233–7.
6. Parmar C, Meda KP. Achilles tendon rupture associated with combination therapy of levofloxacin and steroid in four patients and a review of the literature. Foot Ankle Int 2007;28(12):1287–9.
7. Holmes GB, Lin J. Etiologic factors associated with symptomatic Achilles tendinopathy. Foot Ankle Int 2006;27:952–9.
8. Paavola M, Kannus P, Jarvinen TA, et al. Achilles tendinopathy. J Bone Joint Surg Am 2002;84:2062–76.
9. Monto RR. Platelet rich plasma treatment for chronic Achilles tendinosis. Foot Ankle Int 2012;33(5):379–85.
10. Schepsis AA, Jones H, Haas AL. Achilles tendon disorders in athletes. Am J Sports Med 2002;30:287–305.
11. Lykoudis EG, Contodimos GV, Ristanis S, et al. One-stage complex Achilles tendon defect reconstruction with an Achilles tendon allograft and a gracilis free flap. Foot Ankle Int 2010;31(7):634–8.
12. Kvist MH, Lehto MU, Josza L, et al. Chronic Achilles paratenonitis: an immunohistologic study of fibronectin and fibrinogen. Am J Sports Med 1988;16:616–23.
13. Coughlin MJ, Schon L. Disorders of tendons. In: Mann RA, Coughlin MJ, Saltzman CL, editors. Surgery of the foot and ankle, vol. 1, 8th edition. Philadelphia: Mosby Elsevier; 2007. p. 1149–277.
14. Johnston E, Scranton P Jr, Pfeffer GB. Chronic disorders of the Achilles tendon: results of conservative and surgical treatments. Foot Ankle Int 1997;18(9):570–4.

15. Reddy SS, Pedowitz D, Parekh S, et al. Surgical treatment for chronic disease and disorders of the Achilles tendon. J Am Acad Orthop Surg 2009;17:3–14.
16. Ortmann FW, McBryde AM. Endoscopic bony and soft-tissue decompression of the retrocalcaneal space for the treatment of Haglund deformity and retrocalcaneal bursitis. Foot Ankle Int 2007;28:149–53.
17. Metcalfe D, Achten J, Costa ML. Glucocorticoid injections in lesions of the Achilles tendon. Foot Ankle Int 2009;30(7):661–5.
18. Garras DN, Raikin SM, Bhat SB, et al. MRI is unnecessary for diagnosing acute Achilles tendon ruptures: clinical diagnostic criteria. Clin Orthop Relat Res 2012;470(8):2268–73.
19. Keating JF, Will EM. Operative versus non-operative treatment of acute rupture of tendo Achillis: a prospective randomised evaluation of functional outcome. J Bone Joint Surg Br 2011;93(8):1071–8.
20. Henríquez H, Muñoz R, Carcuro G, et al. Is percutaneous repair better than open repair in acute Achilles tendon rupture? Clin Orthop Relat Res 2012;470(4):998–1003.
21. Patel A, Ogawa B, Charlton T, et al. Incidence of deep vein thrombosis and pulmonary embolism after Achilles tendon rupture. Clin Orthop Relat Res 2012;470(1):270–4.
22. Porter DA, Mannarino FP, Snead D, et al. Primary repair without augmentation for early neglected Achilles tendon ruptures in the recreational athlete. Foot Ankle Int 1997;18:557–64.
23. Wapner KL, Pavlock GS, Hecht PJ, et al. Repair of chronic Achilles tendon rupture with flexor hallucis longus tendon transfer. Foot Ankle 1993;14:443–9.
24. Rahm S, Spross C, Gerber F, et al. Operative treatment of chronic irreparable Achilles tendon ruptures with large flexor hallucis longus tendon transfers. Foot Ankle Int 2013;34(8):1100–10.
25. Kearney RS, Costa ML. Collagen-matrix allograft augmentation of bilateral rupture of the Achilles tendon. Foot Ankle Int 2010;31(6):556–9.

Plantar Heel Pain

Andrew J. Rosenbaum, MD[a],*, John A. DiPreta, MD[a],
David Misener, BSc(HK), CPO, MBA[b]

KEYWORDS

- Plantar heel pain • Plantar fascia • Plantar fasciitis • Windlass mechanism
- Heel spur • Baxter nerve • First branch lateral plantar nerve
- Extracorporeal shock-wave therapy

KEY POINTS

- Approximately 1 in 10 people are predicted to develop such heel pain during their lifetime.
- Plantar fasciitis is the most common cause of plantar heel pain and is responsible for 80% of the cases.
- Plantar heel pain is usually responsive to conservative interventions, including home stretches, nonsteroidal antiinflammatory drugs, orthoses, night splints, and, at times, corticosteroid injections and extracorporeal shock-wave therapy.
- If conservative measures do not provide pain relief, surgery can be considered.

INTRODUCTION

Plantar heel pain is a very common complaint that can cause significant discomfort and disability. Approximately 1 in 10 people are predicted to develop such heel pain during their lifetime, with more than 2 million individuals undergoing treatment of it annually in the United States.[1,2] Although 1% of all visits to orthopedic surgeons are attributed to heel pain, it is also commonly treated by internists and family practitioners.[3] The annual cost of the evaluation and treatment of plantar heel pain by these providers is estimated at approximately $284 million.[4]

The cause, diagnosis, and effective management of plantar heel pain have challenged practitioners since the early 1800s, when Wood first described plantar fasciitis, citing an infectious origin.[5] In the 1930s, gonorrhea, syphilis, tuberculosis, and streptococcal infections were thought to be responsible.[6] The focus then shifted to plantar fat pad impingement by heel spurs.[7] A plethora of conditions are now acknowledged as causes of plantar heel pain.

A thorough history and physical examination are crucial to the diagnosis of plantar heel disorders. Although plantar fasciitis is the most common culprit, accounting for

[a] Division of Orthopaedic Surgery, Albany Medical College, 255 Patroon Creek Boulevard, Apartment 1214, Albany, NY 12206, USA; [b] Clinical Prosthetics and Orthotics, 149 South Lake Avenue, Albany, NY 12208, USA
* Corresponding author.
E-mail address: Andrewjrosenbaum@gmail.com

Med Clin N Am 98 (2014) 339–352
http://dx.doi.org/10.1016/j.mcna.2013.10.009
0025-7125/14/$ – see front matter © 2014 Elsevier Inc. All rights reserved.
medical.theclinics.com

80% of patients with inferior heel pain, the clinician's differential must always include other causes. Mechanical, rheumatologic, and neurologic conditions can all manifest as plantar heel pain. This article reviews the relevant anatomy and biomechanics of the plantar hindfoot, the cause of plantar heel pain, pertinent components of the physical examination, useful diagnostic adjuncts, as well as both conservative and operative treatment modalities.

ANATOMY OF THE PLANTAR FASCIA AND HINDFOOT

The plantar fascia is a broad fibrous aponeurosis that spans the plantar surface of the foot (**Fig. 1**). It originates from the medial and anterior aspects of the calcaneus and helps to divide the intrinsic plantar musculature of the foot into 3 distinct compartments: medial, central, and lateral. Distally, the plantar fascia forms 5 digital bands at the metatarsophalangeal joints. Each digital band then divides to pass on either side of the flexor tendons, inserting into the periosteum at the base of the proximal phalanges.

The plantar fascia has a continuous connection with the Achilles tendon, leading to tightening of the plantar fascia when tensile loads are applied to the tendon. For this reason, Achilles tendon stretching and night splinting have become effective conservative treatments for plantar fasciitis.

The heel's fat pad, first described by Teitze in 1921, is also an integral component of the plantar hindfoot.[8] It is anchored to both the calcaneus and skin, acting as a shock absorber for the hindfoot. It helps to dissipate impact forces caused by heel strike during ambulation, which generates forces up to 110% of one's body weight when walking and 250% of body weight when running.[9] However, after 40 years of age, it begins to degenerate, losing some of its overall thickness and height. With this deterioration, softening and thinning of the fat pad occur, which leads to diminished protection of the heel.[10]

BIOMECHANICS OF THE PLANTAR FASCIA AND HINDFOOT

The foot and its ligaments can be thought of as a truss, with the calcaneus, midtarsal joint, and metatarsals forming the truss's medial longitudinal arch.[11] The plantar fascia acts as a tie-rod, preventing arch collapse via its great tensile strength, particularly during weight bearing. Preservation of the medial longitudinal arch is crucial for ambulation in a systematic and efficient manner. With arch collapse, the appropriate timing of pronation and supination during the gait cycle is altered, leading to inefficient foot function.

The *windlass mechanism* is a term used to describe the role of the plantar fascia in dynamic function during gait; a windlass is the tightening of a rope or cable.[12] As one's toes are dorsiflexed, the plantar fascia tightens, shortening the distance between the calcaneus and metatarsals and elevating the medial longitudinal arch (**Fig. 2**).[13] In the high-arched position, less tension on the truss is required for arch support, as opposed to a low-arched position. In other words, in a high-arched position, there is less tension on the plantar fascia.

CAUSE OF PLANTAR HEEL PAIN

A multitude of mechanical, neurologic, and rheumatologic conditions can manifest as plantar heel pain (**Box 1**). The mechanical causes include derangements of the plantar fascia, calcaneal stress fractures, and heel pad disorders. Although heel spurs are intimately associated with these conditions, they do not directly cause plantar heel

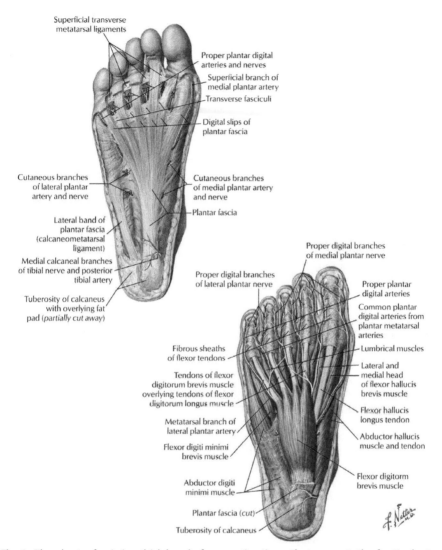

Fig. 1. The plantar fascia is a thick band of connective tissue that supports the foot's plantar arch. It originates at the calcaneal tuberosity of the hindfoot, ultimately inserting into the periosteum at the base of the toes' proximal phalanges. (Netter illustration from www.netterimages.com. © Elsevier Inc. All rights reserved.)

pain. Neurologic disorders are typically caused by nerve compression, whereas rheumatoid conditions may present with systemic manifestations. Infection, which was once thought to be the primary cause of heel pain, is not as common as previously thought.

Fascial derangements include rupture and fasciitis. Rupture most often occurs acutely following trauma or athletic competition, whereas plantar fasciitis is a subacute and degenerative process resulting from repetitive and excessive loading of the fascia.

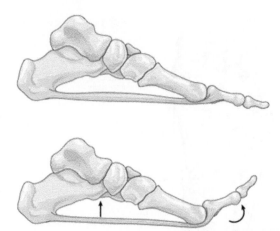

Fig. 2. The windlass mechanism occurs with dorsiflexion of the toes, which leads to tightening of the plantar fascia. (*From* Greisberg J. Foot and ankle anatomy and biomechanics. In: DiGiovanni CW, Greisberg J, editors. Core knowledge in orthopedics: foot and ankle. Philadelphia: Elsevier; 2007; with permission.)

After the metatarsals, the calcaneus is the most common location in the foot for a stress fracture.[14] These injuries most frequently occur in those with osteopenia of the calcaneus and athletes involved in running and jumping sports. Both benign and malignant neoplasms can also cause plantar heel pain. Benign lesions include simple bone cysts, which can weaken bone and cause pathologic fracture. Malignant lesions include primary tumors, of which Ewing sarcoma is the most common, and metastatic disease, including endometrial adenocarcinoma, bronchogenic carcinoma, bladder cancer, and gastric cancer.[15–18]

The deterioration of the fat pad's structural integrity, with advancing age and weight gain, is also thought to contribute to heel pain. Although some think that the progressive thinning of the fat pad is primarily responsible, others have shown an increased thickness to correlate most closely with pain. Further, some think that a reduced elasticity, not fat pad thickness, is the most significant factor.[10,19] Prichasuk[20] found that pad elasticity was reduced in those with pain and that elasticity decreases with increasing age and body weight.

Heel spurs are often associated with heel pain; up to 75% of patients with pain have been shown to have spurs (**Fig. 3**).[21–23] However, spurs are also common in those

---

Box 1
The differential diagnosis of plantar heel pain

- Plantar fasciitis
- Fat pad atrophy
- Partial or complete plantar fascial rupture
- Calcaneal stress fracture
- Plantar nerve impingement
- Hindfoot deformity (cavus or calcaneus)
- Inflammatory enthesopathy

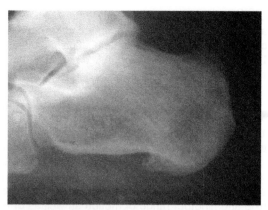

Fig. 3. Lateral radiograph of the hindfoot. A heel spur is evident on the inferior aspect of the calcaneus. (*From* Berkson EM, Greisberg J, Theodore GH. Heel pain. In: DiGiovanni CW, Greisberg J, editors. Core knowledge in orthopedics: foot and ankle. Philadelphia: Elsevier; 2007; with permission.)

without heel pain, suggesting that they are not necessarily the cause of pain.[23] In a randomly chosen sample of 1000 patients, Shmokler and colleagues[21] found a 13.2% incidence of heel spurs but only a 5.2% incidence of heel pain. This finding suggests that both spurs and pain may develop from a common underlying pathologic condition. The work of Kumai and Benjamin[24] supports this notion because their cadaveric study identified degenerative changes within the plantar fascia as the cause of spur formation.

HISTORY AND PHYSICAL EXAMINATION

A comprehensive history is imperative when evaluating patients with plantar heel pain. The patients' general health and past medical history must be reviewed first, identifying any prior treatments for plantar heel pain (ie, medications, injections, therapy, orthoses, surgeries) and the presence of comorbidities. Obesity is an independent risk factor for the development of plantar fasciitis and is present in up to 70% of patients with this disorder.[25,26] It is also important to ask about constitutional symptoms, such as weight loss, fevers, chills, and night sweats, which are findings that suggest a neoplastic or infectious process.

The clinician should inquire into patients' recreational and occupational activities because work-related weight bearing, like obesity, is an independent risk factor for plantar fasciitis.[25] When discussing athletics, the specific sport being played can help differentiate the diagnosis because those who perform running and jumping activities are particularly vulnerable to plantar heel pain. It is also helpful to determine if the pain occurs during heel strike as opposed to push off; if it occurs at the onset of, during, or after activity; and the type of shoe and its insole being used when the pain is present.

A description of the pain and its alleviating and exacerbating factors will assist the clinician in establishing a diagnosis. With the exception of an acute hindfoot fracture or plantar fascia rupture, patients will typically describe the pain as gradual in onset. Of note, those patients with a plantar fascia rupture often have histories of corticosteroid injection.[27,28] Pain that is worse with the first steps in the morning or when standing after prolonged sitting is consistent with plantar fasciitis. These patients may also experience decreased pain with progressive activity, only to have it return later in the day. Constitutional symptoms in the setting of night and/or rest pain suggest either a neoplastic or infectious process. Bilateral plantar heel pain, particularly in conjunction with joint pain and pain at multiple sites of tendon/ligament insertion, suggests that the pain may be related to a rheumatologic process, such as ankylosing spondylitis or Reiter syndrome. With nerve entrapment, patients may describe burning, tingling, or numbness.[29,30]

The physical examination is another critical component of the workup because determination of the location of the pain will facilitate the proper diagnosis. The examination includes a visual assessment of the foot, which may identify swelling, skin breakdown, bruising, or deformity. Palpation of the foot's bony prominences and tendinous insertions near the heel and midfoot must also be done, noting any defects or tenderness; Achilles tendon tightness can contribute to the pain. Observation of ankle and hindfoot range of motion as well as of the foot's posture and arch during weight bearing should also be performed. The physician should also evaluate the patients' spine because an L5-S1 radiculopathy can cause plantar heel pain.

With proximal plantar fasciitis, tenderness over the medial aspect of the calcaneal tuberosity is present. Conversely, distal plantar fasciitis produces pain in the distal aspect of the plantar fascia. Passive dorsiflexion of the toes exacerbates the pain in both the proximal and distal types because this stretches the entire plantar fascia. When a rupture of the plantar fascia occurs, a palpable defect may be evident at the calcaneal tuberosity, along with localized swelling and ecchymosis.[31] Findings suggestive of plantar fibromatosis include pain along the plantar fascia in conjunction with palpable nodules.

A calcaneal stress fracture is diagnosed on physical examination by the squeeze test in which diffuse heel pain is elicited with medial and lateral heel compression. Swelling and warmth may also be present. Neoplastic processes must be considered in the setting of persistent heel pain that is refractory to conservative treatment.

Tarsal tunnel syndrome is a compression neuropathy involving the posterior tibial nerve as it traverses the tunnel. Percussion of the nerve within the tarsal tunnel, as well as simultaneous dorsiflexion and eversion, may reproduce symptoms, which include pain and numbness that radiate to the plantar heel. The findings seen with plantar fasciitis are often similar. However, unlike tarsal tunnel syndrome, patients with plantar fasciitis will have pain with passive toe dorsiflexion. Patients may also present with entrapment of the first branch of the lateral plantar nerve (Baxter nerve, FBLPN). Because of its close proximity to the medial calcaneal tubercle, it is usually present with plantar fasciitis and difficult to distinguish.

Pain that is attributed to the fat pad is centered more proximally than the plantar fascia's origin. It is often associated with erythema and inflammation at the plantar heel. On palpation, it is often softened and flattened.

DIAGNOSTIC ADJUNCTS

The history and physical examination will often reliably diagnose the cause of plantar heel pain. However, when the diagnosis remains unclear, imaging modalities and laboratory studies can be obtained. Plain radiographs provide information about the foot's bony structures and alignment. Weight-bearing anteroposterior and lateral views are standard, with axial and 45° medial oblique views included at times. Heel spurs are commonly seen on the lateral radiographs of patients with plantar heel pain (see **Fig. 3**). A calcaneal lucency, referred to as the *saddle sign* often accompanies the spur, visible just proximal to it on the radiograph.[19] Although soft tissues are poorly visualized on plain radiographs, tumors, osteomyelitis, stress fractures, and fat pad atrophy are sometimes visible.

When a calcaneal stress fracture is suspected, a triple-phase bone scan will have increased uptake. With plantar fasciitis, this too will occur.[32,33] However, the increased uptake in this setting will be localized to the inferomedial aspect of the heel, enabling this test to distinguish the two processes.

Magnetic resonance imaging (MRI) has become a frequently used adjunct in the evaluation of plantar heel pain because it provides great detail of soft tissue structures through its multiplanar capability. Fascial thickening and increased signal intensity within the plantar fascia are typical MRI findings seen with plantar fasciitis. Admittedly, these findings are nonspecific, making MRI most useful for excluding other causes of heel pain. It has been shown that plantar fibromatosis, tumors, infection, and nerve entrapment are all reliably diagnosed with MRI.[34,35]

Ultrasound can identify fascial thickenings and soft tissue edema in the plantar heel and is becoming a commonly used diagnostic tool. In the setting of plantar fasciitis, ultrasound will reveal thickened, hypoechoic fascia. Although the quality of images obtained is operator dependent, some studies suggest that it is superior to MRI, with fat pad edema and degeneration being detected earlier via this modality. Ultrasound is also inexpensive and fast, further distinguishing it from MRI.[36]

When bilateral or recalcitrant heel pain is present, clinicians should order a complete blood count, erythrocyte sedimentation rate, rheumatoid factor, antinuclear antibodies, uric acid, and human leukocyte antigen-B27 studies. These tests may help identify a rheumatologic or autoimmune disorder, such as a seronegative spondyloarthropathy, Behçet syndrome, or inflammatory bowel arthritis.

Nerve conduction velocity and electromyography testing can objectively delineate the severity of a compression neuropathy around the foot and ankle as well as diagnose a spinal radiculopathy or peripheral neuropathy. However, these studies are of more benefit in the diagnosis of tarsal tunnel syndrome than plantar nerve entrapment because the FBLPN is difficult to examine with these tests.[37]

TREATMENT OF PLANTAR HEEL PAIN
Conservative Modalities

Mechanical, rheumatologic, and neurologic sources of plantar heel pain require, and are usually responsive to, a trial of conservative measures. Interventions include home stretching programs and physical therapy, nonsteroidal antiinflammatory drugs (NSAIDs), injections, heel pads, orthoses, night splints, and extracorporeal shockwave therapy (ESWT). In a work by Wolgin and colleagues,[38] 82 of 100 patients' plantar heel pain improved with conservative therapy, and an additional 15 patients were able to work and perform activities despite having mild symptoms. Callison[39] found that 73% of patients treated with nonoperative modalities had significant improvement within 6 months of treatment, whereas only 20% failed to improve.[39] A study by Davies and colleagues[40] also supports nonoperative interventions because they showed that less than 50% of patients who had a surgical procedure for heel pain were completely satisfied with the results.

A home stretching program is the first-line treatment of plantar heel pain. Both plantar fascia–specific and Achilles tendon–based protocols are available. Plantar fascia–specific stretching attempts to recreate the windlass mechanism, whereas Achilles tendon programs attempt to optimize the length of the gastrocnemius-soleus complex. DiGiovanni and colleagues[41] compared these protocols and showed that heel pain was resolved or improved at 8 weeks in 52% of patients treated with a plantar fascia–specific program versus 22% of those performing Achilles tendon exercises. However, at the 2-year follow-up, no difference was evident between the two groups.[41]

NSAIDs are an appropriate treatment of plantar heel pain but are typically prescribed in conjunction with another intervention, such as stretching. The true effectiveness of NSAIDs is, thus, unclear because they are infrequently the sole treatment modality. Although up to 76% of patients report successful outcomes with their use, no study to date has examined their efficacy alone.[38]

Corticosteroid injections are a commonly used treatment of plantar fasciitis, with one study identifying 170 of 233 orthopedic surgeons polled as using steroid injections for heel pain.[42] However, there is limited evidence to suggest that this intervention is effective at providing sustained pain relief. Crawford and colleagues[43] found improved symptoms at 1 month but not at 6 months as compared with a control group. Complications of steroid injection include rupture of the plantar fascia and fat pad atrophy.[27] One's injection technique can reduce the incidence of these complications; the needle should be placed superior to the fascia, from the medial side. This placement spreads the solution across the fascial layer, avoiding the fat pad and plantar nerves.

The injection of botulinum toxin A (BTX-A) is also being used to treat plantar foot pain. Its analgesic and antiinflammatory properties make it an intriguing intervention. In a placebo-controlled, double-blinded study, Babcock and colleagues[44] associated BTX-A injections with significant improvements in pain relief and foot function at both 3 and 8 weeks following treatment. Elizondo-Rodriguez and colleagues[45] have also found BTX-A to be an effective treatment of plantar fasciitis. In their prospective, randomized, double-blinded, and controlled clinical trial, the effectiveness of BTX-A injected into the gastrocnemius-soleus complex was compared with steroid injection into the medial plantar fascia. Over the 6 months that the patients were followed after receiving one of the two aforementioned injections, the group who received the BTX-A was found to have faster and more sustained symptom relief.[45]

Heel pads, foot orthoses, and shoe modifications are adjunctive modalities often used in the treatment of plantar heel pain. From a biomechanical perspective, foot orthoses are designed to place the foot and lower extremity in a more advantageous position by minimizing the existing stresses to the static and dynamic soft tissues of the foot and lower limb; orthoses off-load the plantar fascia, recreate the shape of the heel pad, and decrease excessive pronation.[46–48]

Commonly used orthoses include prefabricated silicone or rubber heel cups and arch supports, felt pads, custom arch supports, the University of California Biomechanics Laboratory orthosis (UCBL), and the supramalleolar ankle foot orthosis (SMO). The UCBL shoe insert is a maximum control foot orthotic that was named after the location in which it was developed, the University of California Berkeley Laboratory in 1967 (Fig. 4). It has since been defined as a deep-seated foot orthosis. The UCBL differs from other foot orthoses in that it fully encompasses the heel, which in turn holds the heel, or hindfoot, in a neutral, vertical position. While correcting and holding the heel in a neutral position, the UCBL also controls the inside arch of the foot and the outside border of the forefoot. These 3 corrective forces keep the foot held in a neutral position.

The SMO, as with other orthoses, gets its name for the part of the body for which it encompasses (Fig. 5). This orthosis supports the leg just above the medial and lateral malleoli. The SMO is designed to maintain a vertical or neutral heel while also supporting the 3 arches of the foot, which can help improve standing balance and walking. This design also allows for more control of the ankle and foot. It is more supportive than a UCBL but less supportive than a standard ankle foot orthosis (AFO).

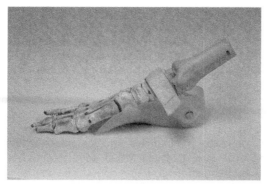

Fig. 4. The UCBL orthosis. (*Courtesy of* David Misener, BSc, CPO, MBA, Albany, NY.)

Shoes are integral to the success of an orthosis because they help to stabilize the orthosis within the shoe and around the foot. A proper shoe provides stability and shock absorption. How a shoe is built also makes a difference in its fit and function. Neutral-arched feet should be placed in shoes with firm midsoles, straight to semi-curved lasts, and moderate hindfoot stability. Low-arched or flat feet should be placed in shoes with a straight last and with motion control to help stabilize the feet. High-arched feet require cushioning and moderate hindfoot stability to compensate for the lack of natural shock absorption.

Ample evidence exists based on subjective pain relief, symptom resolution, and patient satisfaction for the success of orthosis.[49] In a randomized study by Pfeffer and colleagues,[2] 236 patients were randomized into 5 treatment groups: 1 control and 4 with different shoe inserts. Those treated with prefabricated inserts had the largest improvement in heel pain.[2] Roos and colleagues[50] also found foot orthoses to be effective in both the short- and long-term treatment of plantar fasciitis. In this prospective randomized trial, those who used orthoses experienced a 62% decrease in pain at 1 year as compared with patients treated with night splints. Admittedly, other studies have questioned the effectiveness of foot orthoses, identifying only small benefits.[51] Despite this, heel pads and orthoses are powerful tools in the clinician's armamentarium for the treatment of plantar heel pain.

Night splints are designed to prevent shortening of the plantar fascia during long periods of rest, with the goal of alleviating morning start-up pain. The night splint AFO

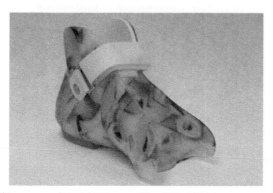

Fig. 5. The SMO. (*Courtesy of* David Misener, BSc, CPO, MBA.)

should be placed in 5° of dorsiflexion. Wapner and Sharkey[52] reported that 11 of their 14 patients improved when splinted in this position. Conversely, Probe and colleagues[53] found no significant benefit in adding night splinting to a standard NSAID and stretching protocol. Casting has also been used to unload the heel and immobilize the plantar fascia, hoping to reduce the repetitive microtrauma associated with plantar fasciitis.

ESWT is indicated for patients who have had at least 6 months of plantar fasciitis heel pain recalcitrant to at least 3 nonsurgical interventions (**Fig. 6**). The powerful shock waves break up scar tissue, stimulate angiogenesis, promote new bone formation, disrupt calcific deposits, and increase cytokine diffusion. Good or excellent results in the setting of chronic heel pain have been reported in 57% to 80% of patients.[54,55] ESWT is often performed under conscious sedation with regional anesthesia. It is well tolerated by patients. The contraindications include patients with hemophilia, coagulopathies, malignancy, and skeletal immaturity.

OPERATIVE TREATMENT

Surgery is indicated in the treatment of plantar heel pain that has failed a minimum of 6 months of conservative modalities (**Box 2**). An open partial release of the plantar fascia is the standard intervention. Although both open and endoscopic techniques have been described, there is no consensus as to the best choice; no studies have been conducted that directly compare these two techniques. Because entrapment neuropathy of the FBLPN presents similarly to plantar fasciitis, decompression of this nerve is frequently performed concurrently. Watson and colleagues[56] reported that 93% of their patients had satisfactory outcomes with partial medial plantar fasciectomy and nerve decompression. When nerve decompression is to be performed, an open approach is advocated because the risk of nerve injury may be higher with endoscopic procedures.[57]

Resection of heel spurs is also performed at times, most commonly in conjunction with the aforementioned procedures. However, Manoli and colleagues[58] reported calcaneal fractures secondary to extensive resection, an unwelcome complication of this procedure. Additionally, the notion that the subcalcaneal spur is the cause of plantar pain has lost popularity in recent years; therefore, this supplementary procedure is being performed less frequently. Fallat and colleagues[59] retrospectively compared percutaneous plantar fasciotomy with open fasciotomy and heel spur resection, determining that the percutaneous procedure

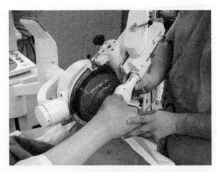

Fig. 6. ESWT. (*From* Berkson EM, Greisberg J, Theodore GH. Heel pain. In: DiGiovanni CW, Greisberg J, editors. Core knowledge in orthopedics: foot and ankle. Philadelphia: Elsevier; 2007; with permission.)

Box 2
Algorithm for the treatment of plantar fasciitis

If history and physical examination consistent with plantar fasciitis, begin

- Home stretching program multiple times daily (either plantar fascia specific or Achilles tendon stretching)
- Wear shoes with good support and a premade or custom-made orthotic
- Trial of NSAIDs

If no improvement

- Reexamine patient and consider alternative diagnoses
- If still consistent with plantar fasciitis, add alternative treatment, such as night splints and corticosteroid injection

If symptoms persist more than 6 months

- Consider shock-wave therapy
- Consider surgery

---

was as effective at relieving the plantar fasciitis pain and that those patients had a faster return to full activity.

Gastrocnemius recession is another procedure that may be indicated for the treatment of plantar fasciitis recalcitrant to conservative interventions. Because limited ankle dorsiflexion, specifically isolated gastrocnemius contracture, is frequently associated with plantar fasciitis, the release of the gastrocnemius can be an effective treatment.[60] Abbassian and colleagues[61] found proximal medial gastrocnemius release to provide complete or significant pain relief in 81% of their patients treated with this. Additionally, none of their patients reported worsening of their symptoms.

SUMMARY

Plantar heel pain is a frequently encountered phenomenon that transcends multiple medical specialties, including orthopedic surgery and primary care. Plantar fasciitis is the most common cause. However, other mechanical, rheumatologic, neurologic, and infectious causes exist; a comprehensive history and physical examination is pivotal to making the correct diagnosis. When the cause remains unclear after the evaluation, diagnostic adjuncts are available and include triple-phase bone scan, MRI, ultrasound, and laboratory studies. Regardless of diagnosis, nonoperative interventions are the mainstay of treatment and include but are not limited to stretching, NSAIDs, orthoses, and steroid injections. Operative intervention is only indicated after 6 months of failed conservative modalities.

REFERENCES

1. Crawford F, Atkins D, Edwards J. Interventions for treating plantar heel pain. Cochrane Database Syst Rev 2000;(3):CD000416.
2. Pfeffer G, Bacchetti P, Deland J. Comparison of custom and prefabricated orthoses in the initial treatment of proximal plantar fasciitis. Foot Ankle Int 1999; 20(4):214–21.
3. Riddle DL, Schappert SM. Volume of ambulatory care visits and patterns of care for patients diagnosed with plantar fasciitis: a national study of medical doctors. Foot Ankle Int 2004;25(5):303–10.

4. Tong KB, Furia J. Economic burden of plantar fasciitis treatment in the United States. Am J Orthop 2010;39(5):227–31.

5. Leach RE, Seavey MS, Salter DK. Results of surgery in athletes with plantar fasciitis. Foot Ankle 1986;7(3):156–61.

6. Chang CC, Miltner LJ. Periostitis of the os calcis. J Bone Joint Surg 1934;16: 355–64.

7. DuVries HL. Heel spur (calcaneal spur). Arch Surg 1957;74:536–42.

8. Pfeffer GB. Plantar heel pain. In: Myerson MS, editor. Foot and ankle disorders. Philadelphia: WB Saunders; 2000. p. 834–50.

9. Perry J. Anatomy and biomechanics of the hindfoot. Clin Orthop Relat Res 1983;(177):9–15.

10. Jahss MH, Kummer F, Michelson JD. Investigations into the fat pads of the sole of the foot: heel pressure studies. Foot Ankle 1992;13:227–32.

11. Hicks JH. The mechanics of the foot. II. The plantar aponeurosis and the arch. J Anat 1954;88(1):25–30.

12. Viel E, Esnault M. The effect of increased tension in the plantar fascia: a biomechanical analysis. Physiother Pract 1989;5:69–73.

13. Kwong PK, Kay D, Voner PT, et al. Plantar fasciitis: mechanics and pathomechanics of treatment. Clin Sports Med 1988;7:119–26.

14. Narvaez JA, Narvaez J, Ortega R, et al. Painful heel: MR imaging findings. Radiographics 2000;20:333–52.

15. Berlin SJ, Mirkin GS, Tubridy SP. Tumors of the heel. Clin Podiatr Med Surg 1990; 7:307–21.

16. Cooper JK, Wong FL, Swenerton KD. Endometrial adenocarcinoma presenting as an isolated calcaneal metastasis. A rare entity with good prognosis. Cancer 1994;73:2779–81.

17. Bergqvist D, Mattsson J. Solitary calcaneal metastasis as the first sign of gastric cancer. A case report. Ups J Med Sci 1978;83:115–8.

18. Kaufmann J, Schulze E, Hein G. Monarthritis of the ankle as manifestation of a calcaneal metastasis of bronchogenic carcinoma. Scand J Rheumatol 2001;30:363–5.

19. Amis J, Jennings L, Graham D, et al. Painful heel syndrome: radiographic and treatment assessment. Foot Ankle 1988;9:91–9.

20. Prichasuk S. The heel pad in plantar heel pain. J Bone Joint Surg Br 1994;76: 140–2.

21. Shmokler RL, Bravo AA, Lynch FR, et al. A new use of instrumentation in fluoroscopy controlled heel spur surgery. J Am Podiatr Med Assoc 1988;78:194–7.

22. Snook GA, Chrisman OD. The management of subcalcaneal pain. Clin Orthop Relat Res 1972;82:163–8.

23. Williams PL, Smibert JG, Cox R, et al. Imaging study of the painful heel syndrome. Foot Ankle 1987;7:345–9.

24. Kumai T, Benjamin M. Heel spur formation and the subcalcaneal enthesis of the plantar fascia. J Rheumatol 2002;29:1957–64.

25. Riddle DL, Pullsic M, Pidcoe P, et al. Risk factors for plantar fasciitis: a matched case-control study. J Bone Joint Surg Am 2003;85:872–7.

26. Tahririan MA, Motififard M, Tahmasebi MN, et al. Plantar fasciitis. J Res Med Sci 2012;17:799–804.

27. Acevedo JI, Beskin JL. Complications of plantar fascia rupture associated with corticosteroid injection. Foot Ankle Int 1998;19(2):91–7.

28. Sellman JR. Plantar fascia rupture associated with corticosteroid injection. Foot Ankle Int 1994;15(7):376–81.

29. Schepsis AA, Jones H, Haas AL. Achilles tendon disorders in athletes. Am J Sports Med 2002;30:287–305.
30. Kinoshita M, Okuda R, Morikawa J, et al. The dorsiflexion-eversion test for diagnosis of tarsal tunnel syndrome. J Bone Joint Surg Am 2001;83-A: 1835–9.
31. Ahstrom JP Jr. Spontaneous rupture of the plantar fascia. Am J Sports Med 1988;16:306–7.
32. Graham CE. Painful heel syndrome: rationale of diagnosis and treatment. Foot Ankle 1983;3(5):261–7.
33. Sewell JR, Black CM, Chapman AH, et al. Quantitative scintigraphy in diagnosis and management of plantar fasciitis (calcaneal periostitis): concise communication. J Nucl Med 1980;21(7):633–6.
34. Theodorou DJ, Theodorou SJ, Resnick D. MR imaging of abnormalities of the plantar fascia. Semin Musculoskelet Radiol 2002;6(2):105–18.
35. Farooki S, Theodorou DJ, Sokoloff RM, et al. MRI of the medial and lateral plantar nerves. J Comput Assist Tomogr 2001;25(3):412–6.
36. Kamel M, Eid H, Mansour R. Ultrasound detection of heel enthesitis: a comparison with magnetic resonance imaging. J Rheumatol 2003;30(4):774–8.
37. Baxter DE, Pfeffer GB. Treatment of chronic heel pain by surgical release of the first branch of the lateral plantar nerve. Clin Orthop Relat Res 1992;(279):229–36.
38. Wolgin M, Cook C, Graham C, et al. Conservative treatment of plantar heel pain: long-term follow-up. Foot Ankle Int 1994;15(3):97–102.
39. Callison WI. Heel pain in private practice [abstract]. Presented at the Orthopaedic Foot Club. Dallas (TX), April 4, 1989.
40. Davies MS, Weiss GA, Saxby TS. Plantar fasciitis: how successful is surgical intervention? Foot Ankle Int 1999;20(12):803–7.
41. DiGiovanni BF, Nawoczenski DA, Malay DP, et al. Plantar fascia–specific stretching exercise improves outcomes in patients wlth chronic plantar fasciitis: a prospective clinical trial with two-year follow-up. J Bone Joint Surg Am 2006;88: 1775–81.
42. Fadale PD, Wiggins ME. Corticosteroid injections: their use and abuse. J Am Acad Orthop Surg 1994;2(3):133–40.
43. Crawford F, Atkins D, Young P, et al. Steroid injections for heel pain: evidence of short-term effectiveness. A randomized controlled trial. Rheumatology 1999;38: 974–7.
44. Babcock MS, Foster L, Pasquina P, et al. Treatment of pain attributed to plantar fasciitis with botulinum toxin A: a short-term, randomized, placebo-controlled, double-blind study. Am J Phys Med Rehabil 2005;84:649–54.
45. Elizondo-Rodriguez J, Araujo-Lopez Y, Moreno-Gonzalez JA. A comparison of botulinum toxin A and intralesional steroids for the treatment of plantar fasciitis: a randomized, double-blinded study. Foot Ankle Int 2013;34:8–14.
46. Heiderscheit B, Hamill J, Tiberio D. A biomechanical perspective: do foot orthoses work? Br J Sports Med 2001;35(1):4–5.
47. Kogler GF, Veer FB, Solomonidis SE, et al. The influence of medial and lateral placement of orthotic wedges on loading of the plantar aponeurosis. J Bone Joint Surg Am 1999;81(10):1403–13.
48. Nester CJ, van der Linden ML, Bowker P. Effect of foot orthoses on the kinematics and kinetics of normal walking gait. Gait Posture 2003;17(2):180–7.
49. Gross ML, Davlin LB, Evanski PM. Effectiveness of orthotic shoe inserts in the long-distance runner. Am J Sports Med 1991;19(4):409–12.

50. Roos E, Engstrom M, Soderberg B. Foot orthoses for the treatment of plantar fasciitis. Foot Ankle Int 2006;27:606–11.
51. Landorf KB, Keenan AM, Herbet RD. Effectiveness of foot orthoses to treat plantar fasciitis: a randomized trial. Arch Intern Med 2006;166:1305–10.
52. Wapner KL, Sharkey PF. The use of night splints for treatment of recalcitrant plantar fasciitis. Foot Ankle 1991;12:135–7.
53. Probe RA, Baca M, Adams R, et al. Night splint treatment for plantar fasciitis: a prospective randomized study. Clin Orthop Relat Res 1999;(368):190–5.
54. Helbig K, Herbert C, Schostok T, et al. Correlations between the duration of pain and the success of shock wave therapy. Clin Orthop Relat Res 2001;(387): 68–71.
55. Rompe JD, Schoellner C, Nafe B. Evaluation of low-energy extracorporeal shock wave application for treatment of chronic plantar fasciitis. J Bone Joint Surg Am 2002;84:335–41.
56. Watson TS, Anderson RB, Davis WH, et al. Distal tarsal tunnel release with partial plantar fasciotomy for chronic heel pain: an outcome analysis. Foot Ankle Int 2002;23(6):530–7.
57. Neufeld SK, Cerrato R. Plantar fasciitis: evaluation and treatment. J Am Acad Orthop Surg 2008;16:338–46.
58. Manoli A 2nd, Harper MC, Fitzgibbons TC, et al. Calcaneal fracture after cortical bone removal. Foot Ankle 1992;13(9):523–5.
59. Fallat LM, Cox JT, Chahal R, et al. A retrospective comparison of percutaneous plantar fasciotomy and open plantar fasciotomy with heel spur resection. J Foot Ankle Surg 2013;52:288–90.
60. Patel A, DiGiovanni B. Association between plantar fasciitis and isolated contracture of the gastrocnemius. Foot Ankle Int 2011;32:5–8.
61. Abbassian A, Kohls-Gatzoulis J, Solan MC. Proximal medial gastrocnemius release in the treatment of recalcitrant plantar fasciitis. Foot Ankle Int 2012;33: 14–9.

Outpatient Assessment and Management of the Diabetic Foot

John A. DiPreta, MD

KEYWORDS

- Diabetes mellitus • Peripheral neuropathy • Charcot arthropathy • Ulceration

KEY POINTS

- Patients with diabetes are at risk for the development of peripheral neuropathy.
- Peripheral neuropathy, when associated with a traumatic event, can lead to Charcot (neuropathic) arthropathy.
- Charcot arthropathy often leads to significant deformity of the ankle and hindfoot.
- Deformity due to neuropathic arthropathy when associated with the insensate foot puts the patient at significant risk for ulcer formation.
- Neuropathic changes in the foot and ankle are best initially managed with immobilization. This immobilization protects the foot from injury, allowing for the process to develop while minimizing further progression.
- For unstable deformities or neuropathic ulcers, surgical correction of these deformities may be required. Urgent referral should be made to the foot and ankle specialist for those individuals with an ulcer or in whom Charcot arthropathy is suspected.

INTRODUCTION

Diabetes is characterized by high blood glucose. Individuals with high blood sugars fall into one of 2 categories. Type I diabetes is characterized by an inability to manufacture insulin due to autoimmune destruction of the insulin-producing pancreatic beta cells.[1] It represents approximately 5% of all diagnosed cases of diabetes. Exogenous insulin is necessary for survival. It typically is first diagnosed in children and young adults. Risk factors included autoimmune, genetic, or environmental causes. Type II diabetes accounts for 95% of diagnosed diabetes in adults. A well-balanced diet along with exercise and certain prescription medications can help control complications. Diabetes is a major cause of heart disease, vision loss, kidney failure, and lower extremity amputation. The final common pathway to limb loss is peripheral neuropathy, peripheral vascular disease, ulceration, and

Division of Orthopaedic Surgery, Albany Medical Center, Albany Medical College, Capital Region Orthopaedics, 1367 Washington Avenue, Suite 200, Albany, NY 12206, USA
E-mail address: jamddipreta@netscape.net

Med Clin N Am 98 (2014) 353–373
http://dx.doi.org/10.1016/j.mcna.2013.10.010
medical.theclinics.com
0025-7125/14/$ – see front matter

infection. Tight glucose control, as measured by A1C levels, can help prevent these complications.[2]

From 1990 through 2010, the number of new cases of diagnosed diabetes nearly tripled. This rise in incidence is attributed to increases in obesity, decreases in physical activity, and an aging US population.[3] The prevalence during this same time period also increased, and many people are unaware of their undiagnosed diabetes. It is thought that if trends continue, as many as 1 in 3 American adults will have diabetes by 2050.[4]

Medical expenses for a person with diabetes are more than twice as high as those without diabetes. In 2007, the estimated cost of diabetes in the United States was $174 billion. This included $116 billion in direct medical care costs and $58 billion in costs due to disability, productivity loss, and premature death.[5]

The ability to lead a functional life hinges on one's mobility. Managing the sequelae of diabetic foot disease (peripheral neuropathy, Charcot arthropathy, and peripheral vascular disease) is thus essential.

The focus of this review is to define the various manifestations of peripheral neuropathy, the pathophysiology of foot ulceration, neuropathic arthropathy (Charcot arthropathy), their assessment, and initial steps in management. Criteria for referral to an orthopedic foot and ankle surgeon are also discussed.

PATHOGENESIS OF INSULIN-DEPENDENT DIABETES MELLITUS

Insulin-dependent diabetes mellitus (IDDM) is most common in individuals of Northern European descent and less common in African American, Native American, and Asian individuals. These differences may be explained by varied genetic susceptibility in racially distinct populations; however, diet and environmental factors likely play a role.[6] Susceptibility is inherited, and the main gene associated with a predisposition to IDDM is the major histocompatibility complex (MHC) on chromosome 6 in the region associated with the genes encoding for HLA recognition molecules. The interaction to a cell bearing an HLA molecule associated with an antigenic peptide and a T lymphocyte bearing a receptor capable of recognizing the HLA peptide complex triggers the activation and proliferation of T lymphocytes. Susceptibility or resistance to IDDM is associated with different HLA-DR and HLA-DQ genotypes, and 95% of patients with IDDM has at least 1 of these HLA-DR antigens.[1]

IDDM is a chronic autoimmune disease that exists in a preclinical phase. The most consistent histologic finding of the pancreas is the lack of insulin-secreting beta cells. Associated with this is a chronic inflammatory infiltrate. Histologic studies have suggested that an 80% reduction in the volume of beta cells is necessary to induce symptomatic IDDM.[7]

The association of microvascular disease and neuropathy with diabetes and the relationship of these conditions to the duration of diabetes suggest that they are linked to hyperglycemia. The Diabetes Control and Complications Trial (DCCT) demonstrated that the incidence and development of retinopathy, nephropathy, and neuropathy could be reduced by intensive treatment.[2]

The retina, kidney, and nerves are freely permeable to glucose. Increases in blood glucose concentrations leads to increased intracellular concentration of both glucose and its metabolic by-products. The mechanism by which hyperglycemia leads to microvascular and neurologic complications includes the increased accumulation of polyols through the aldose reductase pathway and of advanced glycosylation end products.[8]

PERIPHERAL NEUROPATHY

Diabetic neuropathy is one of the most common complications of diabetes mellitus and has many clinical presentations. The intensity and the functional and anatomic abnormalities parallel the degree and duration of hyperglycemia. It is the chronic hyperglycemia that leads to the loss of myelinated and unmyelinated fibers, Wallerian degeneration, and blunted nerve fiber production. Proposed mechanisms for these changes include the formation of sorbitol by aldose reductase and the formation of advanced glycosylation end products. Thus, treatment is directed at optimization of blood glucose levels. In the DCCT,[1] intensive treatment decreased the occurrence of clinical neuropathy by 60%.[2]

Peripheral neuropathy can be broadly classified in 3 ways: sensory, motor, and autonomic. Each type will manifest itself into distinct patterns, and it is these patterns that contribute to the complications that can occur in the diabetic patient. The practitioner must suspect that neuropathy will be present in all patients with type 2 diabetes and in patients with type 1 diabetes of more than 5 years' duration. A single type of neuropathy may exist in isolation or, more commonly, in combination with the other neuropathies.

Sensory neuropathy can be classified as distal symmetric polyneuropathy, focal neuropathy, and diabetic amyotrophy. Motor neuropathies may be defined by the muscles that are involved. Associated with motor neuropathy are predictable patterns of foot deformities that put the patient at risk for ulceration. Autonomic neuropathy is classified by the system that is affected. In particular, this relates to the sudomotor function that controls sweat production in the feet.

In sensory nerve involvement, the nerves with the longest axons are affected first. This leads to the classic "stocking-and-glove" distribution. Large fiber damage results in diminished vibratory sensation, position sense, muscle strength, sharp dull discrimination, and 2-point discrimination. Diabetic amyotrophy is an uncommon variant of somatic neuropathy that is predominantly motor in nature and affects the proximal muscles of the lower extremities. Its clinical presentation is similar to a muscular dystrophy. In sensorimotor neuropathy, it is important to ask about recent falls, balance problems, and gait disturbances. In addition, assessing for loss of Achilles tendon and patellar reflexes is important.

Distal symmetric polyneuropathy is the most common form of diabetic neuropathy. It is associated with variable pain, motor disturbance, nerve palsies, ulcerations, burns, gangrene, and Charcot arthropathy.[9]

Motor neuropathy can manifest itself by affecting the intrinsic musculature of the foot. This results in unopposed function of the extrinsic muscles, which leads to clawing of the toes. This clawing creates a significant mechanical imbalance that puts the diabetic foot at risk for ulceration.

Autonomic neuropathy affects both sympathetic and parasympathetic function. Sympathetic dysfunction can be seen with abnormal neurogenic blood flow. This is thought also to play a role in the development of neuropathic arthropathy. Sudomotor neuropathy may cause hyperhidrosis in the upper extremities and anhidrosis in the lower extremities. The skin of the lower extremities may feel pruritic and display thinning, hair loss, dryness, flaking, cracks, and increased callus formation. These skin changes put the patient at risk for ulceration and ultimately infection.

Neuropathy has a lifetime prevalence of approximately 25% to 50% in those with diabetes.[10] Complications from diabetic neuropathy account for 50% to 75% of nontraumatic amputations.[11] Although frequent screening of diabetic patients reduces the risk of lower extremity amputations, reversing existent diabetic neuropathy is difficult to achieve.[12]

Pathogenesis

Proposed mechanisms to the development of diabetic neuropathy include nonenzymatic glycosylation, increases in oxidative stress, neuroinflammation, and activation of the polyol and protein kinase C (PKC) pathways.[12]

Advanced glycosylation end products (AGEs) are formed in an irreversible fashion as glucose becomes incorporated into proteins. AGE receptors on macrophages induce monocytes and endothelial cells to increase production of inflammatory cytokines and adhesion molecules. This increased inflammatory response may lead to vascular permeability and procoagulant activity. Patients with this type of neuropathy complain of pain and stiffness throughout their bodies. The neuropathic pain may be diffuse and not localized to the hands and the feet.

The polyol pathway activates increasing intracellular levels of fructose and sorbitol. Neither of these products can easily exit cells, and thus create an osmotic gradient leading to water penetration of proteins, and in peripheral nerves this leads to axonal edema and alteration of nerve function. Peripheral nerves become increasing sensitive to light touch and patients will have hyperalgesia on examination.

The protein kinase C pathway activation affects renal blood flow as well as vascular contractility and permeability. Activation of this pathway has been most closely linked to retinopathy and neuropathy.

In response to hyperglycemia, cellular mitochondria activate superoxide production, amplifying the cytotoxic effects induced by other pathogenic pathways. Oxidative stress appears to be triggered more as a result of postprandial fluctuations of blood glucose than with sustained hyperglycemia.

The production of free radicals and superoxide leads to activation of microglial cells, which in turn produce inflammatory cytokines, further damaging neural structures and altering their activity. **Fig. 1** is a schematic representation of the effects of hyperglycemia on the biochemical pathways leading to diabetic neuropathy.

Assessment

The highest rates of neuropathy in patients with type 2 diabetes occur in those who have hyperglycemia for longer than 25 years. In these individuals, it is important to identify modifiable and nonmodifiable risk factors that contribute to the hyperglycemia and, thus, neuropathy. In doing so, there is an opportunity to intensify management or possibly eliminate an individual's progression toward long-term neuropathic complications. Examples of modifiable risk factors include obesity, smoking, hyperglycemia (elevated Hb A1C), and hypertension. Nonmodifiable risk factors include age, family history, and duration of diabetes.[12]

A routine history and neurologic examination are essential when screening diabetic patients thought to be at risk for neuropathy. This is a critical step, as it is neuropathy that leads to the devastating complications associated with it. The neuropathic pain experienced by the patient is chronic, progressive, and serves no protective function. Minimal stimuli may lead to hyperalgesic symptoms. In addition to the structural and mechanical imbalances it creates (Charcot arthropathy, ulceration), it also contributes to depression and sleep disturbances.[12] The clinical evaluation should include the following:

1. Careful inspection of the foot. It is important to assess for skin turgor, ulceration, and deformity. Dry skin in combination with deformity and neuropathy is a significant risk factor for ulceration.

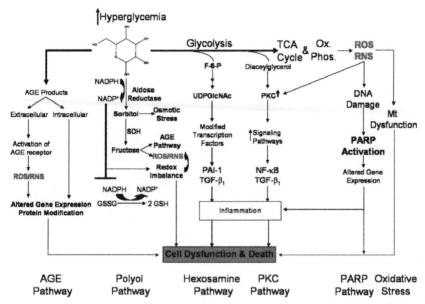

Fig. 1. A schematic representation of the effects of hyperglycemia on the biochemical pathways leading to diabetic neuropathy. (*From* Edwards JL, Vincent AM, Cheng HT, et al. Diabetic neuropathy: mechanisms to management. Pharmacol Ther 2008;120:1–34; with permission.)

2. Evaluate ankle reflexes, as this indicates advanced peripheral neuropathy.
3. Check for proprioception. Move the hallux up or down with the patient's eyes closed and determine the patient's ability to determine direction.
4. Check for allodynia and hyperalgesia. Using a cold stimulus or a vibrating 128-Hz tuning fork may elicit allodynia.
5. Determine protective sensation. Using a Semmes-Weinstein 5.07 monofilament (Northcoast Medical, Gilroy, CA), check for sensation in areas of pressure, considered to be at risk for ulceration (**Fig. 2**).

Once it is established that an individual has diabetic neuropathy, follow-up is essential. In a patient with neuropathy but no mechanical deformities, visits with the primary care physician on a routine basis is appropriate. An individual with deformity or with a history of or a current ulcer needs more frequent follow-up, and an urgent referral to the appropriate foot and ankle specialist is critical.

The varied mechanisms for neuropathic changes in the diabetic patient pose potential targets for pharmacotherapeutic treatment. Although few options to reverse the root causes exist, the readers are referred to a review of therapeutic strategies in the medical management of diabetic neuropathy.[13]

The American Orthopedic Foot and Ankle Society has recommendations that can be viewed in the "Patient Section" at www.aofas.org. Suggested care for patients includes inspection of their feet on a daily basis for ulcers, blisters, and skin irritations. They should never walk barefoot or in flip-flops or sandals. They should call their physician for any injuries or disruptions in their skin. Shoes should be purchased at the end of the day and should not be "broken in." Patients should avoid paring or trimming calluses on their own, leaving it a medical professional. Nail and toe care should be focused on trimming nails straight across and avoiding chemical agents on corns and calluses.

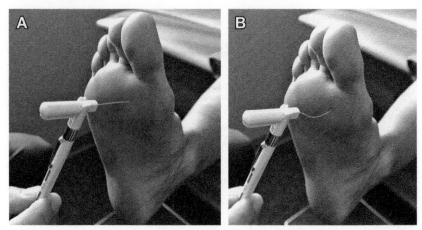

Fig. 2. Demonstration of the assessment of peripheral neuropathy using the Semmes-Weinstein monofilament: (*A*) depicts application of the monofilament, (*B*) demonstrates the bend in the filament when assessing for neuropathy.

CHARCOT ARTHROPATHY

Charcot arthropathy is a progressive deterioration of weight-bearing joints, typically in the foot and ankle in patients with diabetic peripheral neuropathy. In 1868, Jean Marie Charcot described this pattern of bone destruction in patients with tabes dorsalis. Involvement of the knee was commonly associated with syphilis. The first description of neuroarthropathy occurring in conjunction with diabetes was described in 1936.

There are believed to be 2 general causes of neuropathic arthropathy. One is termed the neurotraumatic theory, the other being the neurovascular theory. The neurotraumatic theory is based on the repetitive microtrauma and ensuing bony dissociation and destruction that occurs in the foot that is insensate and lacks proprioception. The neurovascular causes are believed to be due to autonomic dysfunction leading to hyperemia and osteopenia, which effectively weakens and allows progressive destruction in the setting of ongoing trauma. Muscle imbalance in combination with joint stiffness creates eccentric forces and high pressures on the foot, setting the stage for ulceration. The initial bony dissolution and dissociation leads to ligamentous laxity and the supporting structures of the foot become completely compromised. A common pattern seen is a rocker-bottom deformity, which is essentially a reversal of the normal foot architecture. Up to 50% of those individuals with a Charcot foot can recall an injury or an inciting event. Such events may include a twisting injury to the foot or the ankle, or it may occur subsequent to a procedure on the foot (**Fig. 3**).

Neuropathic arthropathy may be seen in up to 10% patients with neuropathy and up to 35% of those affected will have bilateral involvement. It is typically encountered in patients with poorly controlled diabetes and in those who have had the disease for more than 10 years.[14] **Fig. 3** represents the summary of events that lead to the Charcot foot.

The clinical appearance of the foot will vary based on the stage of presentation. Eichenholtz[15] was credited with the description of the clinical stages of the disease. Stage I is considered the fragmentation stage, and is what is typically seen in the acute stages. This is characterized by radiographic evidence of periarticular erosion and joint dislocation. Patients may present earlier with warmth, erythema, and swelling of the foot before the onset of deformity. It often has the appearance of an infection. Stage II represents the coalescence phase, whereby the bony changes begin to

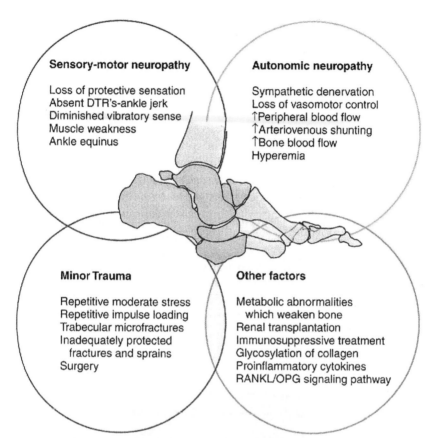

Sensory-motor neuropathy

Loss of protective sensation
Absent DTR's-ankle jerk
Diminished vibratory sense
Muscle weakness
Ankle equinus

Autonomic neuropathy

Sympathetic denervation
Loss of vasomotor control
↑Peripheral blood flow
↑Arteriovenous shunting
↑Bone blood flow
Hyperemia

Minor Trauma

Repetitive moderate stress
Repetitive impulse loading
Trabecular microfractures
Inadequately protected
   fractures and sprains
Surgery

Other factors

Metabolic abnormalities
   which weaken bone
Renal transplantation
Immunosuppressive treatment
Glycosylation of collagen
Proinflammatory cytokines
RANKL/OPG signaling pathway

Fig. 3. Representation of the summary of events that lead to the development of a neuropathic foot deformity. *Abbreviations:* DTR, deep tendon reflexes, OPG, osteoprotegerin. (*From* Sanders LJ, Frykberg RG. The Charcot foot. In: Bowker JH, Pfeifer MA, editors. Levin and O'Neal's the diabetic foot. 7th edition. Philadelphia: Elsevier; 2008. p. 257–83; with permission.)

stabilize and there is resorption of bony debris. Stage III is the consolidation or reparative phase and represents the stage at which the foot deformity becomes stable (**Fig. 4**). The foot is often deformed, but progression has ceased. Recognition of this process in its earliest stages is critical to optimize intervention and to prevent the long-term sequelae.

Radiographically and anatomically, Charcot arthropathy can be characterized. In its atrophic form, osteolysis occurs in the distal metatarsals, localizing it to the forefoot (**Fig. 5**). Hypertrophic Charcot is localized to the midfoot, hindfoot, or ankle, and it is this form that is classified by the Eichenholtz scheme.

Brodsky[16] described 3 types of Charcot arthropathy based on the involvement of the anatomic location of the foot. Type 1 involves the midfoot and leads to plantar and medial prominences. Type 2 involves the transverse tarsal joint and leads to the greatest instability of the hindfoot. Type 3 has 2 subparts: 3A involves the ankle joint, which also is characterized by instability and prolonged bone healing, and 3B is a pathologic fracture of the calcaneus creating a wide heel and a flat foot.[17] **Fig. 6** demonstrates the geographic radiographic appearance of the Charcot foot.

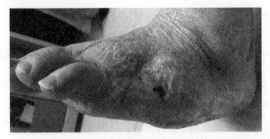

Fig. 4. Clinical appearance of a 49-year-old man with a midfoot neuropathic foot deformity.

The diagnosis of Charcot is largely a clinical one based on the physician's suspicion and the clinical presentation of the patient. When a neuropathic patient demonstrates bone and joint abnormalities, the diagnosis of Charcot arthropathy must be suspected. Distinguishing an acute Charcot process from osteomyelitis can be very challenging. The diagnosis hinges on a detailed history, thorough examination of the foot and ankle, and initial radiographic studies. Use of magnetic resonance imaging (MRI) can be equivocal when trying to distinguish Charcot arthropathy from osteomyelitis. Osteomyelitis should be presumed when there is chronic soft tissue ulceration and infection contiguous to bone. However, in the case of Charcot arthropathy, noninfectious soft tissue inflammation accompanies progressive bone and joint destruction in a well-vascularized, neuropathic, nonulcerated foot.[18] Bone biopsy should be reserved for those individuals in whom the diagnosis remains ambiguous.

Computed tomography, MRI, and technetium scans have limitations in distinguishing between Charcot arthropathy and osteomyelitis. Leukocyte scanning with

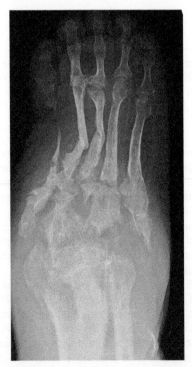

Fig. 5. Anteroposterior (AP) radiograph depicting a forefoot neuropathic deformity.

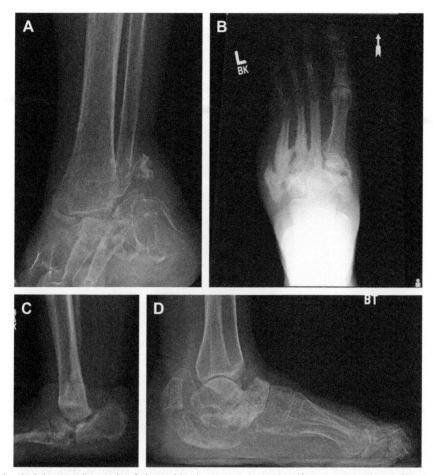

Fig. 6. (*A*) AP radiograph of the ankle demonstrating a hindfoot neuropathic deformity. There is dislocation of the calcaneus under the talus where it is resting under the fibula. (*B*) AP radiograph of a patient with neuropathic changes of the tarsometatarsal joints. (*C*) Lateral radiograph of the ankle demonstrating absence of the talus and dissolution of the hindfoot. (*D*) Lateral radiograph of the foot depicting neuropathic changes of the calcaneus demonstrating rocker bottom appearance.

Indium-111 has been shown to have high specificity and negative predictive value for osteomyelitis.[19] It has also been noted that 111-In labeled leukocytes do not accumulate in neuropathic bone.

When the diagnosis of Charcot arthropathy has been established, management is based on the stage of presentation to the practitioner and the presence or absence of infection. The goal of treatment is to maintain a stable, plantigrade foot so as to prevent ulceration. Optimal treatment for the Charcot foot is prevention. Risk assessment and stratification help identify those at risk: individuals in the sixth or seventh decade, patients who have had diabetes for more than 10 years, and those with loss of protective sensation. Physical manifestations include swelling, redness, increased skin temperature, and deformity.[20]

Initial management should include elevation to control limb edema, weight-bearing restriction, and, in select individuals, immobilization in a total contact cast (**Fig. 7**).

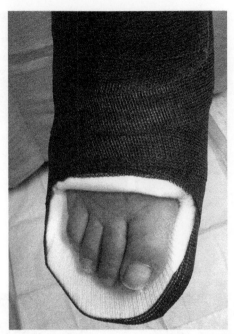

Fig. 7. A total contact cast (TCC). It extends from below the knee and extends past the plantar surface of the toes to provide support and protect the neuropathic foot from further deformity.

Patients who present acutely and are considered candidates for a total contact cast, or those with an ulcer, should be immediately referred to a foot and ankle specialist.

For those who present with deformity and who have passed through the acute phases, customized bracing (**Fig. 8**) and accommodative orthoses (**Fig. 9**) may be considered. Patients should be referred to a foot and ankle specialist or an orthotist experienced with the prescription and/or manufacturing of the appropriate devices. The goal of these devices is to offload prominent areas on the foot and distribute pressure within the shoe in such a way as to minimize risk of ulceration.

The role for use of antiresorptive agents in the management of acute Charcot osteoarthropathy is beginning to emerge; however, their role has yet to be defined.[21] Other emerging technologies include targeting the receptor activator for nuclear factor kappa B ligand (RANKL). RANK is thought to be a critical element in mechanisms controlling osteoclastogenesis and metabolic bone disease.[22]

Surgical intervention is necessary when conservative treatment at offloading and medical optimization have failed to create a stable, plantigrade, ulcer-free foot. Surgical correction is performed when the Charcot process has become quiescent. Surgical intervention typically requires realignment fusions (**Fig. 10**) or, in select cases, primary amputation.

FOOT ULCERATION

The pathophysiology of the development of the diabetic foot ulcer is multifactorial. In combination with the loss of protective sensation that these patients possess, there is

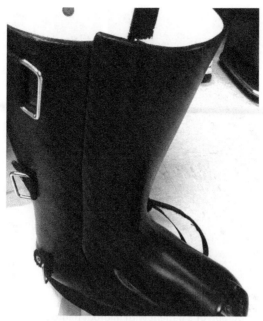

Fig. 8. An accommodative Charcot Restraining Orthotic Walker. It is designed to support the neuropathic foot and can be used when transitioning from a TCC.

a mechanical coupling that increases the risk of development and progression of ulcer formation. Deformity created by Charcot arthropathy, soft tissue contractures, clawing of the toes, and gait abnormality contribute to the mechanical milieu that causes ulceration.

Clawing of the toes is a manifestation of the motor neuropathy that selectively targets the intrinsic muscles of the foot. The deformity created makes the toes vulnerable to ulceration with shoe wear, affecting the plantar and dorsal surfaces of the foot.

Soft tissue contractures, particularly involving the gastrocsoleus complex, are an end result of the advanced glycosylation products causing collagen crosslinking along the length of the entire molecule, causing stiffening of its construct.[23] Altered proprioception and postural instability have been reported in patients with diabetic neuropathy.[24] The loss of afferent feedback during the gait cycle causes increased variability

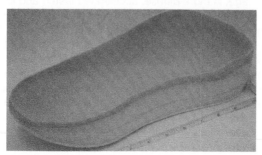

Fig. 9. An accommodative trilayer custom-molded foot insert for a neuropathic foot deformity. The multilayer foam allows for conformity and protection from shear.

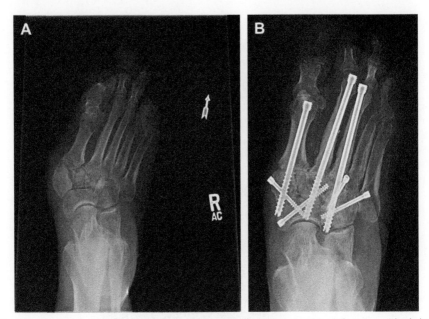

Fig. 10. (*A*) An AP radiograph of a patient with midfoot neuropathic deformity with abduction of the foot that lead to an ulceration. (*B*) Postoperative radiograph of the same patient after undergoing midfoot corrective osteotomy.

of gait kinematics. Additionally, increased plantar flexor moments contribute to abnormal forces contributing to ulcer formation.

The integrity of the skin and the effects of parasympathetic dysfunction compromise the sweat production of the skin. As a result, the skin becomes dry and scaly, and fissures develop. These fissures serve as a portal for infection.

Vascular Disease

Coupled with the mechanical factors that contribute to diabetic foot ulceration is peripheral vascular disease. Primarily ischemic ulcers account for 15% to 20% of foot ulcers, with an additional 15% to 20% due to a mixed neuropathic-vascular etiology.[25] Involvement is most commonly localized to the tibial and peroneal arteries of the calf with sparing of the arteries of the foot.[26] Peripheral vascular disease is more prevalent, occurs at an earlier age, is more diffuse, accelerates faster, and is more extensive in patients with diabetes than in those without diabetes. Plaques develop circumferentially along the length of the vessel and calcification is seen within the tunica media. Additional factors that contribute to atherosclerosis is the dysfunction of nitric oxide. Nitric oxide is a cellular mediator that interferes with monocyte and leukocyte adhesion to the endothelium, platelet-vessel wall interaction, smooth muscle proliferation, and vascular tone. Hyperglycemia, which leads to the formation of superoxides, contributes to this dysfunction, as the reactive oxygen species bind to nitric oxide, limiting its bioavailability.[27]

The assessment of the diabetic patient should include evaluation of pedal pulses. It should be noted that the presence of pulses alone may not be predictive of clinically significant ischemia. Rivers and colleagues,[28] described a cohort of patients who required distal surgical bypass for significant ischemia in the presence of pedal pulses.

In addition to the physical examination, additional noninvasive tests have been used to quantify the severity of peripheral vascular disease. The use of the ankle-brachial index has been used to assess peripheral blood flow. Its validity in patients with diabetes may be less reliable because of the calcification present within the media layer of the distal arteries. The use of systolic toe pressure measurement by photoplethysmography or measuring transcutaneous oxygen tension may be more reliable techniques.[29,30] These measurements are performed in a vascular laboratory and provide an indication of healing potential before consideration of angiography. Arteriography would be considered a "gold standard," but must be instituted with care in this population of people in whom renal disease is often present.[31]

The ankle-brachial index is performed by dividing the segmental ankle systolic pressure by the brachial systolic pressure. Pressure changes typically correlate with flow and an index of 0.5 therefore indicates 50% of expected blood flow. A gradient of 40 mm Hg or greater between segments suggests occlusion or high level of stenosis. The thigh pressure is usually 1.3 times that of the brachial systolic pressure. As noted earlier, the value of ankle pressures may be invalid due to medial calcification. Decreased values, however, can be indicative of significant disease, as no false pressures are likely to occur. Normal indices or elevated pressures should be correlated with toe pressures.[32] The role of toe pressure measurement has been studied. It is felt that absolute toe pressures provide a highly accurate method for determining the likelihood of an ulcer or in minor amputation, thus preventing a more proximal amputation.[33] Toe pressures measuring higher than 40 mm Hg are most predictive of wound healing (**Fig. 11**).

Another method to evaluate the state of limb perfusion, and in particular the skin, is the measurement of transcutaneous partial oxygen pressure. The test is performed by placing a probe over the metatarsal region of the affected foot. After equilibrating the probe to a specific temperature, the oxygen tension of the skin is determined.[34] Although results are difficult to interpret, and may be limited by host and ambient factors, there is support for its use.[30] A transcutaneous oxygen pressure (TCpO2) reading of 40 mm Hg or higher was predictive of adequate perfusion for wound healing in patients undergoing transtibial amputation.[35] In a study by Pinzur and colleagues,[36] healing rates were correlated with TCpO2. The healing rate was 50% with a TCpO2 of 1 to

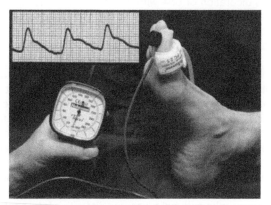

Fig. 11. Clinical photo of measuring toe-pressures. (*From* Hurley JJ. Noninvasive vascular testing in the evaluation of diabetic peripheral arterial disease. In: Bowker JH, Pfeifer MA, editors. Levin and O'Neal's the diabetic foot. 7th edition. Philadelphia: Mosby; 2008. p. 239–55; with permission.)

19 mm Hg, 75% with a TCpO2 of 20 to 29 mm Hg, and 92% at levels higher than 30 mm Hg.

Ulcer Classification

Classification of diabetic foot wounds is important to develop treatment plans, and it is important to communicate with caregivers to monitor progress and outcomes of these lesions. As has been discussed, there are several factors that need to be considered in the assessment and management of these wounds. These factors include perfusion, presence and extent of gangrenous changes, location and severity of vascular disease, location of the ulcer, shape of the ulcer, duration, the presence and depth of infection, infecting organisms, nutritional status, immunosuppression, comorbidities, bony deformity, neuropathy, previous ulcerations, gait disturbances, and abnormal foot pressures.[37] It is through recognition of these factors that we can hopefully intervene, treat, and educate patients so as to minimize risk for amputation and future ulceration.

Approximately 70% to 90% of neuropathic ulcers occur in the forefoot; the heel is the next most common area followed by the midfoot.[17]

Two common classification schemes include the Wagner-Megitt Classification and the Depth Ischemia Classification.

The Wagner-Megitt Classification is known for its simplicity and is often referred to when discussing these lesions. The original system has 6 grades of lesions. The first 4 grades (0, 1, 2 and 3) are based on the physical depth of the lesion involving the soft tissues of the foot. Grades 4 and 5 are based on the extent of lost perfusion in the foot. Most outpatient lesions are grades 0 to 1, whereas grades 2 and 3 ulcers often require hospitalization or surgical intervention. Grades 4 and 5 require amputation and control of residual infection and consideration for further limb revascularization (**Fig. 12**).

The Depth-Ischemia Classification is a modification of the Wagner-Megitt Classification. It makes it easier to distinguish between evaluation of the wound and the vascularity of the foot, which is a limitation of the Wagner-Megitt Classification. Each foot is given a number and letter grade. The number value describes the physical extent of the wound, and the letter grade describes the vascularity. Determination of grade and stage is accomplished with inspection and gentle probing with a blunt, sterile instrument. The grade 0 foot is a foot at risk and represents a foot that has had a previous ulceration or one with characteristics making ulceration likely. A grade 1 lesion is a superficial wound without exposure of deeper structures. Grade 2 lesions are deeper with exposed tendon or joint capsule, with or without infection. Grade 3 lesions are the deepest, with exposed bone and osteomyelitis or abscess (see **Fig. 12**).

Limb perfusion is next determined and assigned letters A, B, C, and D. A grade A foot will demonstrate bounding pedal pulses. These feet do not typically require vascular evaluation or intervention. A grade B foot is the most commonly encountered. It is ischemic but not gangrenous. Lesions of this nature require referral for vascular analysis. Grade C feet have partial gangrene, and grade D feet are completely gangrenous. A vascular evaluation is necessary to determine the level of adequate perfusion, level of potential healing, and the need for revascularization.

Depth-Ischemia Classification is effective at prescribing treatment (**Table 1**). Grade 0 lesions are treated with education, regular visits, and appropriate insoles and shoe wear. Grade 1 lesions require external pressure relief with a total contact cast, bracing, or shoe wear. Grade 2 lesions require surgical debridement, wound care pressure, and antibiotics. Grade 3 lesions require surgical debridement and may require partial ray amputation. Stage A lesions can be observed and followed with regular visits. Stage

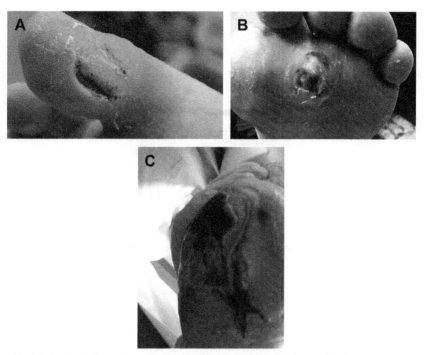

Fig. 12. (*A*) Grade 1 ulceration of hallux. (*B*) Grade 2 ulcer off plantar forefoot with exposed plantar capsule. (*C*) Grade 3 ulcer of calcaneus with necrotic wound bed and exposed calcaneus.

B requires vascular evaluation with possible vascular reconstruction. Stage C requires a proximal or distal bypass and partial amputation. Stage D lesions may require major extremity amputation (transtibial, transfemoral) with vascular reconstruction.[38]

Wound-Healing Strategies

The approach to management of foot lesions is based on the staging, grading, and etiology of the ulcer. This can be accomplished with a combination of mechanical offloading and local wound care.

Offloading can be accomplished through the use of a total contact cast. The application of the cast must be performed by experienced personnel, as serious complications may arise from its use. A patient with a nonhealing ulcer and associated deformity should be referred to a foot and ankle specialist. Other devices that have been described include removable braces and off-loading shoes. These devices, although potentially safer, require patient compliance, which historically has been poor.[39,40]

There is a wide range of wound-healing agents available. This includes, but is not limited to, saline dressings, impregnated gauze, nonadherent dressing, hydrogels, hydrocolloids, calcium alginate, silver, vacuum-assisted closure, and hyperbaric oxygen. The indications for the various agents is vast and the reader is referred to a recent review of the subject.[41]

Local wound debridement, along with application of the previously discussed modalities, are considered for chronic wounds. Office-based debridement is designed to decrease the bacterial burden of the wound. Bacterial overgrowth is a significant

Table 1
The Depth-Ischemia Classification depicting the grading and management of neuropathic foot ulcers

Grade	Definition	Treatment
Depth Classification		
0	The at-risk foot: previous ulcer or neuropathy with deformity that can cause new ulcerations	Patient education: regular examination, appropriate footwear, appropriate insoles
1	Superficial ulceration, not infected	External pressure relief; total-contact cast, walking brace, special footwear, and so forth
2	Deep ulceration exposing a tendon or joint (with or without superficial infection)	Surgical debridement, wound care, pressure relief if the lesion closes and converts to grade 1 (antibiotics as needed)
3	Extensive ulceration with exposed bone and/or deep infection (osteomyelitis) or abscess	Surgical debridement; ray or partial foot amputation; antibiotics; pressure relief if wound converts to grade 1
Ischemia Classification		
A	Not ischemic	None
B	Ischemia without gangrene	Vascular evaluation (eg, Doppler, $tcPo_2$ arteriogram); vascular reconstruction as needed
C	Partial (forefoot) gangrene of the foot	Vascular evaluation; vascular reconstruction (proximal and/or distal bypass or angioplasty); partial foot amputation
D	Complete foot gangrene	Vascular evaluation; major extremity amputation (below knee or above knee) with possible proximal vascular reconstruction

From Brodsky JW. The diabetic foot. In: Coughlin MJ, Mann RA, Saltzman CL, editors. Surgery of the foot and ankle. Philadelphia: Mosby; 2007. p. 1301; with permission.

impediment to wound healing. Enzymatic production by bacteria and the ensuing degradation of fibrin and other growth factors inhibits wound healing. Debridement of dysvascular or necrotic tissue helps decrease the bacterial count and stimulates production of local growth factors.

Finally, additional factors that predict wound healing are a total serum protein concentration of 6.2 g/dL, a serum albumin level of 3.5 g/dL, and a total lymphocyte count of 1500/mm³.[42]

ORTHOTIC MANAGEMENT OF THE DIABETIC FOOT

All too often, institution of an orthotic or an off-loading device is undertaken after someone has healed an ulceration or has undergone a partial foot amputation from an infection created by an ulcer. The goal of a comprehensive diabetic foot program requires communication between the physician and an experienced pedorthist. The goals are to create a protective environment for the foot and to prevent recurrent ulceration.

Improper shoe wear is a common cause of ulcers.[43] There are several objectives for therapeutic shoe wear for the diabetic patient. The shoe should protect the foot from the external environment and relieve areas of pressure and distribute pressure more evenly to minimize risk of ulceration. Shoe wear should protect from shock and shear, especially in cases of significant deformity. Because many feet have significant deformities, it is important to have shoes that accommodate the neuropathic foot.[44]

The key to selecting shoe size is determined by accurately measuring the foot. This should be done both weight bearing and non–weight bearing to determine how much the foot changes. An appropriately sized shoe will have three-eighths to one-half inch between the end of the longest toe and the front of the shoe. The shoe should allow for a small amount of movement of the heel. It is important to educate the patient on proper-fitting shoes.

Foot orthoses are usually prescribed as custom-made devices. The role of the orthosis is to cushion and protect the foot. A well-made orthosis should provide shock absorption and provide shock attenuation. It should provide pressure distribution throughout in cases in which high plantar pressure exists. A total contact design should limit shear and, through the use of soft materials, it should accommodate fixed deformities. A combination of rigid and semirigid material will also limit motion and minimize ulceration.

RECOMMENDATIONS

It is critical that every health professional involved in the care of the diabetic patient take an active role in assessing an individual's risk for foot pathology. The American Diabetes Association recommends that all patients with diabetes receive a thorough foot examination on an annual basis. For patients with a previous ulcer or history of an amputation, screening should be carried out every 3 to 4 months. Patients with active wounds or Charcot arthropathy require more aggressive follow-up with weekly or biweekly visits. This assessment includes observing for protective sensation, foot structure and biomechanical imbalance and limited joint mobility, skin integrity, and vascular status.[45] An assessment of shoe wear also is essential, as improper shoe wear can lead to ulceration. One should maintain a diligent approach in looking for high-risk factors, including advancing age, a history of diabetes for more than 10 years, visual loss, inability to bend, living alone, tobacco use, and risk-taking behavior, in addition to the risk factors discussed previously.[46]

Unfortunately, there are many challenges to the treatment of these diabetic foot problems. Often patients are in denial of their disease and fail to take ownership of their illness and the necessary steps to prevent complications. A screening or prevention program may not effect change in behavior in this patient population. However, in a well-informed and motivated patient, maintaining suggested glucose control is possible through diet, exercise, and medication. It is incumbent for all practitioners to continually educate their patients about the consequences and treatment of diabetes.[47]

Screening patients for risk of ulceration is critical to prevention. Studies have demonstrated the efficacy of such screening, thereby reducing foot ulcers and their consequences.[48,49] Screening helps determine the level of risk and guide additional interventions.[50] Risk assessment is possible based on the history of ulceration, deformity, previous amputation, absence of pedal pulses, and loss of sensation.[50] A patient with risk category 0 who has a normal foot and normal neurovascular function should be educated on daily foot care and shoe wear, and have yearly examinations. A person with risk category 1 demonstrates sensory loss and is advised on daily foot inspection and to obtain soft inlays, and is advised to have the foot examined every 6 months. The patient with a risk category 2 has had a ray amputation, demonstrates sensory loss, and has deformity of the foot. These individuals require more diligent attention with more frequent visits to their physician. Custom-molded inserts are suggested and additional appliances may be necessary to further off-load the forefoot. The patient in risk category 3 has a history of ulceration, deformities, and prior multilevel amputation. These individuals also have diminished or absent pulses. These patients require extensive education and require custom-made accommodative orthoses. External modifications to shoe wear also may be required. Surveillance should be done every 2 months by a qualified health professional. These patients will typically be referred to an orthopedic foot and ankle surgeon to optimize management of the associated deformities.

The individual patient remains the most important player in prevention of foot complications. Through education of the risk factors discussed in the text and physical inspection of the foot, an individual can understand the seriousness of his or her disease. The initial responsibility for management is assigned to the primary care provider. Hopefully, with the information provided in this text, providers will have the necessary background information to understand and assess the diabetic patient at risk for ulceration and amputation and implement the necessary intervention. Any individual with loss of protective sensation, history of ulceration, or prior amputation should be referred to a foot and ankle specialist for treatment. It is important to incorporate family members, when present, into the care of these individuals. This is especially true for patients with poor vision and/or limited mobility, as they cannot adequately monitor their foot skin integrity or changes in their feet.[51] Adherence to guidelines to screening, as put forth by the American Diabetes Association, The American Board of Family Practice, and the Centers for Disease Control and Prevention, can assist the practitioner in caring for these patients with this extremely challenging disease. These recommendations include foot examination at every diabetic visit with screening for risk factors, such as age (older than 40 years), smoking, and duration of diabetes of more than 10 years. Additional recommendations include assessment of ulcer size, plain radiographs, mechanical off-loading, and metabolic control.[52]

REFERENCES

1. Atkinson AM, MacLaren NK. The pathogenesis of insulin dependent diabetes mellitus. N Engl J Med 1994;331(21):1428–36.
2. The Diabetes Control and Complications Trial Research Group. The effect of intensive treatment of diabetes on the development and progression of long term complications in insulin dependent diabetes mellitus. N Engl J Med 1993;339:977–86.
3. Geiss LS, Cowie CC. Type 2 diabetes and persons at high risk for diabetes. In: Narayan KM, Williams D, Gregg EW, et al, editors. Diabetes and public health: from data to policy. New York: Oxford University Press; 2011. p. 15–32.
4. Boyle JP, Thomson TJ, Gregg EW, et al. Projection of the year 2050 Burden of diabetes in the US adult population: dynamic modeling of incidence, mortality and prediabetes prevalence. Popul Health Metr 2010;8:29.
5. Centers for Disease Control and Prevention. National diabetes fact sheet, 2011. Atlanta (GA): Centers for Disease Control and Prevention, US Department of Health and Human Services; 2011. Available at: http://www.cdc.gov/diabetes/pubs/pdf/ndfs_2011.
6. MacLaren N, Atkinson M. Is insulin dependent diabetes mellitus environmentally induced? N Engl J Med 1992;327:348–9.

7. Foulis AK, Liddle CN, Farquharson MA, et al. The histopathology of the pancreas in type 1 (insulin dependent) diabetes mellitus: a 25 year review of deaths in patients under 20 years of age in the United Kingdom. Diabetologia 1986;29:267–74.
8. Clark CM, Lee DA. Presentation and treatment of the complications of diabetes mellitus. N Engl J Med 1995;332:1210–7.
9. Aring AM, Jones DF, Falko JM. Evaluation and prevention of diabetic neuropathy. Am Fam Physician 2005;71:2123–8.
10. Pinart J. Diabetes mellitus and its degenerative complications: a prospective study of 4400 patients observed between 1947 and 1973. Diabete Metab 1977;3:97–107.
11. Vink AI, Mehrabyan A. Understanding diabetic neuropathies. Emerg Med 2004; 5:39–44.
12. Unger J, Cole BE. Recognition and management of diabetic neuropathy. Prim Care 2007;34:887–913.
13. Edwards JL, Vincent AM, Cheng HT, et al. Diabetic neuropathy: mechanisms to management. Pharmacol Ther 2008;120:1–34.
14. Sommer TC, Lee TH. Charcot foot: the diagnostic dilemma. Am Fam Physician 2001;64:1591–8.
15. Eichenholtz SN. Charcot joints. Springfield (IL): Thomas; 1966.
16. Brodsky JW. Outpatient diagnosis and care of the diabetic foot. Instr Course Lect 1993;42:121–39.
17. Laughlin RT, Calhoun JH, Mader JT. The diabetic foot. J Am Acad Orthop Surg 1995;3:218–25.
18. Berendt AR, Lipsky B. Is this bone infected or not? Differentiating neuroarthropathy from osteomyelitis in the diabetic foot. Curr Diab Rep 2004;4(6):424–9.
19. Schauwecker DS. Osteomyelitis: diagnosis with in-111-labelled leukocytes. Radiology 1989;171(1):141–6.
20. Sanders LJ, Frykberg RG. The Charcot foot. In: Bowker JH, Pfeifer MA, editors. Levin and O'Neal's the diabetic foot. 7th edition. Philadelphia (PA): Mosby Elsevier; 2008. p. 257–83.
21. Pitocco D, Riotolo V, Caputo S, et al. Six month treatment with alendronate in acute Charcot neuroarthropathy: a randomized controlled trial. Diabetes Care 2005;28(5):1214–5.
22. Jeffcoate W. Vascular calcification and osteolysis in diabetic neuropathy: is RANKL the missing link? Diabetologia 2004;47(9):1488–92.
23. Guyton GP, Saltzman CL. The diabetic foot: basic mechanisms of disease. J Bone Joint Surg Am 2001;83(7):1084–96.
24. Katoulis EC, Ebdon-Parry M, Hollis S, et al. Postural instability in diabetic neuropathic patients at risk for foot ulceration. Diabet Med 1997;14:296–300.
25. Grunfeld C. Diabetic foot ulcers: etiology, treatment and prevention. Adv Intern Med 1991;37:103–32.
26. Logerfo W, Coffman JD. Vascular and microvascular disease of the foot in diabetes: implications for foot care. N Engl J Med 1984;311:1615–9.
27. Cosentino F, Luscher TF. Endothelial dysfunction in diabetes mellitus. J Cardiovasc Pharmacol 1998;32(Suppl 3):s54–61.
28. Rivers SD, Scher L, Veith FJ. Indications for distal arterial reconstruction in the presence of palpable pedal pulses. J Vasc Surg 1990;12(5):552–7.
29. Apelqvist J, Castenfors J, Larsson J, et al. Prognostic value of systemic ankle and toe blood pressure measurement in outcome of diabetic foot ulcer. Diabetes Care 1989;12:373–8.

30. Ballard JL, Eke CC, Bunt TJ, et al. A prospective evaluation of transcutaneous oxygen measurements in the management of diabetic foot problems. J Vasc Surg 1995;22(4):485–90.
31. Bowering CK. Diabetic foot ulcers: pathophysiology, assessment and therapy. Can Fam Physician 2001;47:1007–16.
32. Hurley JJ. Noninvasive vascular testing in the evaluation of diabetic peripheral arterial disease. In: Bowker JH, Pfeifer MA, editors. Levin and O'Neal's the diabetic foot. 7th edition. Philadelphia: Mosby; 2008. p. 239–55.
33. Holstein P, Noer I, Tonneses KH, et al. Distal blood pressure in severe arterial insufficiency. In: Bergan J, Yao J, editors. Gangrene and severe ischemia of the lower extremities. New York: Gryne and Stratton; 1978. p. 95–114.
34. Aulivola B, Craig RM. Decision making in the dysvascular lower extremity. Foot Ankle Clin 2010;15:391–409.
35. Mustapha NM, Redhead RG, Jain SK, et al. Transcutaneous partial oxygen pressure assessment of the ischemic lower limb. Surg Gynecol Obstet 1983; 156:582–4.
36. Pinzur MS, Sage R, Stuck R, et al. Transcutaneous oxygen as a predictor of wound healing in amputations of the foot and ankle. Foot Ankle 1992;13: 271–2.
37. Brodsky JW. Classification of foot lesions in diabetic patients. In: Bowker JH, Pfeiffer MA, editors. Levin and O'Neal's the diabetic foot. 7th edition. Philadelphia: Mosby; 2008. p. 221–6.
38. Brodsky JW. Outpatient diagnosis and management of the diabetic foot. Instructional course lectures, vol. 42. Rosemont (IL): American Academy of Orthopaedic Surgeons; 1993. p. 121–39.
39. Cavanagh PR, Owings TM. Nonsurgical strategies for healing and preventing recurrence of diabetic foot ulcers. Foot Ankle Clin 2006;11:735–43.
40. Armstrong D, Lavery LA, Kimbriel HR, et al. Activity patterns of patients with diabetic foot ulceration: patients with active ulceration may not adhere to a standard pressure offloading regimen. Diabetes Care 2003;26(9):2595–7.
41. Falanga V. Wound healing and its impairment in the diabetic foot. Lancet 2005; 366(9498):1736–43.
42. Wagner F Jr. A classification and treatment program for diabetic, neuropathic and dysvascular foot problems. Instr Course Lect 1979;28:143–65.
43. Reiber GE, Smith DG, Wallace C, et al. Effect of Therapeutic Footwear on Foot Reulceration in Patients with Diabetes: A Randomized Controlled Trial. JAMA 2002;287(19):2552–8.
44. Janisse DJ, Janisse EJ. Pedorthic and orthotic management of the diabetic foot. Foot Ankle Clin 2006;11:717–34.
45. Mayfield JA, Reiber G, Sanders LJ, et al. Preventive foot care in patients with diabetes. Diabetes Care 1988;21:2161–77.
46. Helfand AE. Assessing and preventing foot problems in older patients who have diabetes mellitus. Clin Podiatr Med Surg 2003;20:573–82.
47. Farber DC, Farber JS. Office based screening, prevention and management of diabetic foot disorders. Prim Care 2007;34:873–85.
48. Singh N, Armstrong DG, Lipsky BA. Preventing foot ulcers in patients with diabetes. JAMA 2005;293:217–8.
49. Willrich A, Pinzur M, McNeil M, et al. Health related quality of life, cognitive function and depression in diabetic patients with foot ulcer or amputation: a preliminary study. Foot Ankle Int 2005;26(2):128–34.

50. Berlet G, Shields N. The diabetic foot. In: Richardson EG, editor. Orthopaedic knowledge update foot and ankle 3. Rosemont (IL): American Academy of Orthopaedic Surgeons; 2004. p. 123–34.

51. Umeh L, Wallhagen M, Nicoloff N. Identifying diabetic patients at high risk for amputation. Nurse Pract 1999;24(8):56–70.

52. Zoorob RJ, Hagen MD. Guidelines on the care of diabetic nephropathy, retinopathy and foot disease. Am Fam Physician 1997;8(56):2021–8.

Index

Note: Page numbers of article titles are in **boldface** type.

Med Clin N Am 98 (2014) 375–389
http://dx.doi.org/10.1016/S0025-7125(14)00023-6
0025-7125/14/$ – see front matter © 2014 Elsevier Inc. All rights reserved.
medical.theclinics.com

Moving?

Make sure your subscription moves with you!

To notify us of your new address, find your **Clinics Account Number** (located on your mailing label above your name), and contact customer service at:

Email: journalscustomerservice-usa@elsevier.com

800-654-2452 (subscribers in the U.S. & Canada)
314-447-8871 (subscribers outside of the U.S. & Canada)

Fax number: 314-447-8029

Elsevier Health Sciences Division
Subscription Customer Service
3251 Riverport Lane
Maryland Heights, MO 63043

*To ensure uninterrupted delivery of your subscription, please notify us at least 4 weeks in advance of move.